Self Appraisal in Laboratory Medicine

MUHAMED T OSMAN

SABIHA PIT

ISBN-10: 1500431737
ISBN-13: 978-1500431730

DEDICATION

This book is dedicated to the students who have been a source of continuous stimulation and to our well wishers in academic arena.
Osman and Sabiha

CONTENTS

PREFACE

With the advent of rapid and amazing advances and recent breakthroughs in various fields of medicine in this millennium, including molecular aspects, genetics, epigenomics, and immunology the literature is inundated with considerable number of books, journals and raving reviews. But regrettably it is rather distressing to note the comparative deficiency of books and guides on evaluation of medical undergraduates pari passu with the magnitude of ever mounting literature on colossal breath taking advances enhancing comprehension of various disciplines of medicine. The relatively alarming dearth of guide books such as this the most useful instruments of evaluation dimensions of embedded knowledge in undergraduate medical students, has prompted publication of this book. This book contains 400 questions in Laboratory Medicine dealing with all important topics of Anatomic Pathology, Chemical Pathology, Hematopathology, Microbiology and Immunology. This will surely serve as an excellent tool for self- appraisal as well as a stimulus for gauging one's abilities to analyze, rationalize and synthesize the knowledge in a manner that would stand in good stead for clinicopathological correlation which is the quintessence of learning Laboratory Medicine. Besides, its systemic use will serve as a barometer for students the subject areas of weakness in which they would benefit from further study. We have taken all efforts to present the answers that will convey adequate useful information. If this is found useful it would confirm our aspirations as not only teachers and trainers but testers as well.

We wish all the readers a salubrious journey through this book which is a compulsory companion to all students. We wish to acknowledge with gratitude all those colleagues who participated in the preparation of this one way or other and particularly students who were the driving force.

Muhamed Osman, PhD and Sabiha Pit, FRCP

1 GENERAL

1.1 General Pathology

1.1.a Questions without answers

1.   The outcomes of acute inflammation include:

    A.   Infarction

    B.   Abscess formation.

    C.   Keloid formation

    D.   Resolution.

    E.   Malignancy

2.   Chemical mediators of acute inflammation include:

    A.   C3

    B.   Leukotrienes

    C.   Corticosteroids

D.   Histamine

E.   Lymphokines.

3.   **Common complications of wound healing include:**

A.   Ischemic effect

B.   formation of excessive granulation tissue

C.   Formation of cancer

D.   Hypertrophic scar

E.   Pathological fractures

4.   **The following are statements regarding granulomatous inflammation:**

A.   Tuberculosis is a common example

B.   It is characterised by epithelioid cells

C.   It arises secondary to presence of foreign body

D.   Caseation necrosis is commonly seen

E.   There is a predominance of neutrophils.

5.   **Cells involved in chronic inflammation include:**

A.   Macrophages

B.   Lymphocytes.

C.   Red blood cells

D.   Epithelioid cells

E.   Endothelial cells

6.   The following are statements regarding thrombus:

A.   The lines of Zahn form a microscopic feature.

B.   Red thrombus is characteristic of arterial thrombosis

C.   Pulmonary embolism is a complication of venous thrombus

D.   It is loosely adherent to vascular endothelium.

E.   Resolution is one of the sequelae

7.   The fate of the thrombus includes:

A.   Recanalisation

B.   Resolution

C.   Deposition of cholesterol

D.   Embolisation

E.   Disseminated intravascular coagulation

8.   Causes of bleeding include:

A.   Aplastic anemia

B.   Vitamin A deficiency

C.   Vitamin K deficiency

D.   Thrombocytosis

E.   Malignancy

9.   **The following are statements regarding hyperpigmentation**

A.   Inflammation is a cause

B.   Many forms of hyperpigmentation are caused by an excess production of melanin.

C.   May occurs due to adrenal insufficiency

D.   May occurs after exposure to certain chemicals such as salicylic acid.

E.   It can sometimes be induced by dermatological laser procedures.

10. **The following are statements regarding calcification:**

A.   It is the accumulation of calcium salts in the body tissue.

B.   Vitamin K deficiency is a cause

C.   Kidney stone is a manifestation.

D.   Metastatic calcification occurs in the gastric mucosa

E.   Metastatic calcification is a systemic elevation of calcium levels in the blood and all tissues.

11. **The following are statements regarding necrosis:**

A.   Gangrenous necrosis is seen in the heart

B.   Liquefactive necrosis is common in the brain

C.   Ischemia is the common cause

D. Protein denaturation is seen in coagulative necrosis

E. Apoptosis is a type of necrosis

12. The following are statements regarding necrosis:

A. Apoptosis is pathological death of cells.

B. Cell injury is associated with a loss of cytosolic calcium

C. Coagulative necrosis is common in the heart

D. Necrosis is usually a result of hypoxic damage.

E. Fatty change in the cells is reversible.

13. The following are statements regarding genetic basis of neoplasia:

A. Mutation of RAS oncogene is frequently seen in human cancers.

B. P53 is a characteristic tumor suppressor gene

C. Retinoblastoma is a malignancy associated with an inherited risk.

D. Genetic studies have no significance in the treatment of cancer.

E. Chromosomal translocations involve large fragments of DNA.

14. The following are statements regarding ischemia:

A. It occurs when the blood supply to a tissue is inadequate to meet the tissue's metabolic demands.

B. Vasculitis is a complication.

C. Arterial emboli to the brain cause ischemic necrosis of brain tissue.

D. Ischemic necrosis of the extremities is a serious problem in the hypertensive patients.

E. Atherosclerosis of the major coronary arteries is responsible for the vast majority of the cases of ischemic heart disease.

15. The following are statements regarding infarction:

A. An infarct is an area of ischemic necrosis.

B. Infarctions often result from sudden reduction of vascular flow by thrombosis or embolism.

C. Infarcts of vital organs are minor causes of mortality.

D. Occasionally, infarction is caused by local vasospasm.

E. Renal artery embolism may infarct the entire kidney.

16. The following are statements regarding dysplasia:

A. It is reversible

B. It occurs before metaplasia

C. Severe dysplasia in most cases is likely to need treatment.

D. The cellular abnormality is not restricted to the originating tissue.

E. Viruses are the most common cause

17. The following are statements regarding metaplasia:

A. It is irreversible

B. The cell of origin for many types of metaplasias is controversial or unknown.

C. Local stem cells become reprogrammed to form a new type of cell.

D. Barrett esophagus is an example of pathological metaplasia

E. Normal physiological metaplasia occurs in endocervix.

18. The following are statements regarding embolism:

A. Arterial embolism can cause vessel occlusion in any part of the body

B. Majority of aortic embolism are clinically silent

C. An embolus landing in the brain from either the heart will likely cause an ischemic stroke.

D. Patients with prosthetic valves carry a significant increase in risk of thromboembolism

E. The main complication of venous embolism is pulmonary embolism

19. The following are statements regarding classification of tumours:

A. Sarcoma   : Cancers derived from epithelial cells

B. Carcinoma : Cancers arising from connective tissue

C. Lymphoma and leukemia   : Cancer arise from hematopoietic cells

D. Germ cell tumor : Cancers derived from pluripotent cells

E. Blastoma   : Cancers derived from immature "precursor" cells

20. **The following are statements regarding grading categories of a tumour:**

   A.   Grade X   :   Grade cannot be assessed

   B.   Grade 1   :   Well differentiated (Low grade)

   C.   Grade 2   :   Moderately differentiated (Intermediate grade)

   D.   Grade 3   :   Poorly differentiated (High grade)

   E.   Geade 4   :   Undifferentiated (High grade)

21. **The following are statements regarding classification of benign tumours:**

   A.   A lipoma is a common benign tumor of fat cells

   B.   A Hamartoma is a benign tumor of cartilage-forming cells

   C.   Adenomas are benign tumors of gland-forming cells

   D.   Teratomas contain many cell types such as skin, nerve, brain and thyroid, because they are derived from germ cells
   E.   A chondroma is a benign tumor that has relatively normal cellular differentiation.

22. **The following are statements regarding wound healing:**

   A.   In the inflammatory phase, bacteria and debris are phagocytosed and removed
   B.   The proliferative phase is characterized by angiogenesis, collagen deposition, granulation tissue formation
   C.   In angiogenesis, new blood vessels are formed by vascular endothelial cells
   D.   In maturation and remodeling phase, the wound is made smaller by the action of myofibroblasts

E.   In the contraction, collagen is remodeled and realigned along tension lines

23.   Systemic factors affecting wound healing include:

A.   Inflammation

B.   Connective Tissue Disorders

C.   Metabolic Diseases

D.   Immunosuppression

E.   Obesity

24.   The following are statements regarding primary intention type of wound healing

A.   It involves epidermis and dermis without total penetration of dermis healing by process of epithelialization

B.   When wound edges are brought together so that they are adjacent to each other.

C.   It maximizes scarring

D.   Most surgical wounds heal by primary intention healing

E.   Well-repaired laceration is an example.

25.   The following are statements regarding metaplasia

A.   It is an adaptation that replaces one type of epithelium with another

B.   It is accompanied by a loss of endothelial function

C.   The cell of origin for many types of metaplasias are unknown

D.   The metaplastic area should be neglected until revised to normal

E.   Barrett's esophagus is an example

26.   The followings are causes of metaplasia:

A.   Cigarette smoke

B.   Bladder stone

C.   Gastro-esophageal reflux

D.   Low pH of vagina

E.   Sleep deprivation

27.   Major pathological microscopic changes of Dysplasia include:

A.   Anisocytosis (cells of unequal size)

B.   Poikilocytosis (abnormally shaped cells)

C.   Hyperchromatism (excessive pigmentation)

D.   Presence of mitotic figures (an unusual number of cells which are currently dividing)

E.   Increased nuclear cytopalsmic ratio

28.   The following are statements regarding dysplasia

A.   It is the earliest form of pre-cancerous lesion.

B.   It is always low grade

C.   It generally consists of an expansion of immature cells

D.   Dysplasia, in which cell maturation and differentiation are delayed, can be contrasted with metaplasia

E.   Myelodysplastic syndrome is an example

29.   The following are statements regarding granuloma

A.   It is a medical term for a tiny collection of immune cells known as macrophages

B.   The macrophages in granulomas are often referred to as "epithelioid"

C.   All granulomas may contain additional cells and matrix, like neutrophils

D.   The difference between granulomas and other types of inflammation is that granulomas form in response to antigens that are resistant to "first-responder" inflammatory cells

E.   The antigen causing the formation of a granuloma is most often an infectious pathogen.

30.   Granulomas are seen in the following diseases:

A.   Tuberculosis

B.   Histoplasmosis

C.   Cat scratch disease

D.   Ulcerative collitis

E.   Sarcoidosis

31.   The following are statements regarding infarction

A.   White infarctions affect solid organs such as the spleen.

B. Severe vasoconstriction is a cause of white infarction

C. Red infarctions generally affect the heart

D. Red infarction affects the small intestine

E. White infarction affects loose tissues that allow blood to collect in the infracted zone

32. The following are statements regarding infarction

A. Myocardial infarction is most commonly due to occlusion of a coronary artery.

B. Cerebral infarction can be atherothrombotic or embolic.

C. Splenic infarction can occur asymptomatically.

D. Limb infarction is presented as leg paralysis

E. Eye infarction can cause sudden visual loss.

33. The following are statements regarding morphological patterns of necrosis:

A. Coagulative necrosis is typically seen in hypoxic environments, such as infarction.

B. Liquefactive necrosis is characterized by the digestion of dead cells to form a viscous liquid mass

C. Fibrinoid necrosis shows amorphous granular debris enclosed within a distinctive inflammatory border.

D. Fat necrosis is specialized necrosis of fat tissue

E. Caseous necrosis is usually caused by immune-mediated vascular damage.

34. Conditions caused by poor calcium absorption:

T   A.   Tartar on teeth

F   B.   Hyper spleenism

T   C.   Arthritic bone spurs

T   D.   Kidney stones

T   E.   Gall stones

35.   Infectious agents are known to be carcinogenic include

A.   Heliobacter pylori   :   MALT lymphoma

B.   HPV virus   :   cervical cancer

C.   Hepatitis B virus   :   liver cancer

D.   EBV virus   :   a type of lymphoma

E.   Schistosoma haematobium   :   bladder cancer

36.   The followings are causes of ischemia:

A.   Atherosclerosis

B.   Hypotention

C.   Sickle cell anemia

D.   Bradycardia

E.   Hypoglycemia

37.   The following are statements regarding malignant tumour:

A.   There is anaplasia of cells

B.   It resembles cell of origin microcopically

C.   Its growth is slow

D.   There is presence of giant cells.

E.   It metastasizes to distant organs

38.   Benign tumours are characterized by

A.   slow growth

B.   absent of capsule

C.   metastasis

D.   different histological pattern from parent tissue

E.   absent of marked necrosis within the tumour

39.   The following are statements regarding chronic inflammation:

A.   Tissue destruction is an important feature

B.   Fibrosis is a common end result.

C.   Granuloma is proliferating blood vessels and fibrous tissue.

D.   Granuloma is common in tuberculosis

E.   Liquefactive necrosis is found at the centre of granulomas.

40.   The following are statements regarding morphologic patterns of inflammation:

A.   Granulomatous inflammation occurs in syphilis.

B.   Fibrinous inflammation is commonly seen in serous cavities.

C.   Purulent inflammation is characteristically occurs due to infection by pyogenic bacteria such as staphylococci infection.

D.   Serous inflammation characterized by the copious effusion of non-viscous serous fluid, commonly produced by mesothelial cells of serous membranes.

E.   Ulcerative inflammation occurs near an epithelium can result in the necrotic loss of tissue from the surface.

41. The following are statements regarding the appearance of granulation tissue:

A.   Light red or dark pink in color, being perfused with new capillary loops or "buds".

B.   Soft to the touch

C.   Moist

D.   Cyst or cavity formation

E.   bumpy (granular) in appearance

42. The following are statements regarding cancer prognosis:

A.   Presence of systemic symptoms has bad prognosis

B.   Site of the tumour does not affect prognosis

C.   Well differentiated tumours have good prognosis

D.   Stage 4 tumours are associated with good prognosis

E.   Responsiveness to therapy has good prognosis

43. Factors that influence development of an infarct include:

A. Dual blood supply and presence of collaterals.

B. Rate of development of vascular obstruction.

C. Tissue vulnerability to hypoxia

D. Tissue metabolic rate.

E. Hypothyroidism.

44. The following are statements regarding an infarct

A. Infarcts are classified on the basis of their size.

B. White infarcts occur with arterial occlusion of solid organs

C. Red infarcts occur with venous occlusions in organs with collateral circulation

D. White infarcts can become hemorrhagic with reperfusion.

E. Red infarcts occur in loose tissues.

45. The following match is true regarding hemorrhage:

A. Chronic blood loss : iron deficiency anemia

B. Thrombocypenia : gum bleeding

C. Car accident with hypovolemia : shock

D. Heamarthrosis : clotting factor deficiency

E. Hematemesis : presence of blood in sputum

46. **Recognized causes of defective neutrophil function include:**

    A. Hepatic failure

    B. Diabetes inspidus

    C. Hodgkins disease

    D. Chediak –higashi syndrome

    E. Renal failure

47. **Causes of cancer include:**

    A. Stress

    B. Genetics

    C. Obesity

    D. Infections

    E. Both ionizing and non-ionizing radiation.

48. **Effects and complications of shock include:**

    A. Adult respiratory distress syndrome

    B. Acute tubular necrosis

    C. Adrenal hyperplasia

    D. Disseminated intravascular coagulation

    E. Heart failure

49. **The following are statements regarding effects of shock:**

A.   Heart failure is a complication in hypovolaemic shock

B.   Circulatory changes in the lung occur when compensatory mechanisms are failing.

C.   Acute ulceration of the stomach and duodenum may complicate shock.

D.   The secretory function of the kidneys is sometimes disturbed in shock

E.   Adrenal haemorrhage occurs occasionally in severe shock.

50.   The following are statements regarding shock:

A.   Cardiogenic shock results from myocardial pump failure caused by intrinsic myocardial damage.

B.   Hypovolemic shock is associated with fractures of bones

C.   Anaphylactic shock initiated by a generalized IgA mediated response.

D.   Cyanotic skin is clinical presentation in cardiogenic shock.

E.   Old age is a factor favoring progression of shock

1.1.b Questions with answers

1.   The outcomes of acute inflammation include:

F   A.   Infarction

T   B.   Abscess formation.

F   C.   Keloid formation

T   D.   Resolution.

F   E.   Malignancy

2.   Chemical mediators of acute inflammation include:

T   A.   C3

T   B.   Leukotrienes

F   C.   corticosteroids

T   D.   Histamine

F   E.   lymphokines.

3.   Common complications of wound healing include:

F   A.   Ischemic effect

T   B.   formation of excessive granulation tissue

F   C.   Formation of cancer

T   D.   hypertrophic scar

F   E.   pathological fractures

4.   The following are statements regarding granulomatous inflammation:

T   A.   Tuberculosis is a common example

T   B.   It is characterised by epithelioid cells

F   C.   It arises secondary to presence of foreign body

T   D.   Caseation necrosis is commonly seen

T   E.   There is a predominance of neutrophils.

5.   Cells involved in chronic inflammation include:

T   A.   Macrophages

T   B.   Lymphocytes.

F   C.   Red blood cells

T   D.   Epithelioid cells

F   E.   Endothelial cells

6.   The following are statements regarding thrombus:

F   A.   The lines of Zahn form a microscopic feature.

F   B.   Red thrombus is characteristic of arterial thrombosis

T   C.   Pulmonary embolism is a complication of venous thrombus

F   D.   It is loosely adherent to vascular endothelium.

T   E.   Resolution is one of the sequelae

7.   The fate of the thrombus includes:

T   A.   Recanalisation

T   B.   Resolution

F   C.   Deposition of cholesterol

T   D.   Embolisation

F   E.   Disseminated intravascular coagulation

8.   Causes of bleeding include:

T   A.   Aplastic anemia

F   B.   Vitamin A deficiency

T   C.   Vitamin K deficiency

F   D.   Thrombocytosis

T   E.   Malignancy

9.   The following are statements regarding hyperpigmentation

T   A.   Inflammation is a cause

T   B.   Many forms of hyperpigmentation are caused by an excess production of melanin.

T   C.   May occurs due to adrenal insufficiency

T   D.   May occurs after exposure to certain chemicals such as salicylic acid.

T   E.   It can sometimes be induced by dermatological laser procedures.

10.   The following are statements regarding calcification:

T   A.   It is the accumulation of calcium salts in the body tissue.

T   B.   Vitamin K deficiency is a cause

T   C.   Kidney stone is a manifestation.

T   D.   Metastatic calcification occurs in the gastric mucosa

T   E.   Metastatic calcification is a systemic elevation of calcium levels in the blood and all tissues.

11.   The following are statements regarding necrosis:

F   A.   Gangrenous necrosis is seen in the heart

T   B.   Liquefactive necrosis is common in the brain

T   C.   Ischemia is the common cause

T   D.   Protein denaturation is seen in coagulative necrosis

F   E.   Apoptosis is a type of necrosis

12.   The following are statements regarding necrosis:

F   A.   Apoptosis is pathological death of cells.

F   B.   Cell injury is associated with a loss of cytosolic calcium

T   C.   Coagulative necrosis is common in the heart

T   D.   Necrosis is usually a result of hypoxic damage.

T   E.   Fatty change in the cells is reversible.

13.   The following are statements regarding genetic basis of neoplasia:

T   A.   Mutation of RAS oncogene is frequently seen in human cancers.

T   B.   P53 is a characteristic tumor suppressor gene

T   C.   Retinoblastoma is a malignancy associated with an inherited risk.

F   D.   Genetic studies have no significance in the treatment of cancer.

T   E.   Chromosomal translocations involve large fragments of DNA.

14.   The following are statements regarding ischemia:

T   A.   It occurs when the blood supply to a tissue is inadequate to meet the tissue's metabolic demands.

F   B.   Vasculitis is a complication.

T   C.   Arterial emboli to the brain cause ischemic necrosis of brain tissue.

F   D.   Ischemic necrosis of the extremities is a serious problem in the hypertensive patients.

T   E.   Atherosclerosis of the major coronary arteries is responsible for the vast majority of the cases of ischemic heart disease.

15.   The following are statements regarding infarction:

T   A.   An infarct is an area of ischemic necrosis.

T   B.   Infarctions often result from sudden reduction of vascular flow by thrombosis or embolism.

F   C.   Infarcts of vital organs are minor causes of mortality.

T   D.   Occasionally, infarction is caused by local vasospasm.

T   E.   Renal artery embolism may infarct the entire kidney.

16.   **The following are statements regarding dysplasia:**

F   A.   It is reversible

F   B.   It occurs before metaplasia

T   C.   Severe dysplasia in most cases is likely to need treatment.

F   D.   The cellular abnormality is not restricted to the originating tissue.

F   E.   Viruses are the most common cause

17.   **The following are statements regarding metaplasia:**

F   A.   It is irreversible

T   B.   The cell of origin for many types of metaplasias is controversial or unknown.

T   C.   Local stem cells become reprogrammed to form a new type of cell.

T   D.   Barrett esophagus is an example of pathological metaplasia

T   E.   Normal physiological metaplasia occurs in endocervix.

18.   **The following are statements regarding embolism:**

T   A.   Arterial embolism can cause vessel occlusion in any part of the body

F   B.   Majority of aortic embolism are clinically silent

T   C.   An embolus landing in the brain from either the heart will likely cause an ischemic stroke.

T   D.   Patients with prosthetic valves carry a significant increase in risk of thromboembolism

T   E.   The main complication of venous embolism is pulmonary embolism

19. The following are statements regarding classification of tumours:

F   A.   Sarcoma   :   Cancers derived from epithelial cells

F   B.   Carcinoma :   Cancers arising from connective tissue

T   C.   Lymphoma and leukemia   :   Cancer arise from hematopoietic cells

T   D.   Germ cell tumor   :   Cancers derived from pluripotent cells

T   E.   Blastoma   : Cancers derived from immature "precursor" cells

20. The following are statements regarding grading categories of a tumour:

T   A.   Grade X   :   Grade cannot be assessed

T   B.   Grade 1   :   Well differentiated (Low grade)

T   C.   Grade 2   :   Moderately differentiated (Intermediate grade)

T   D.   Grade 3   :   Poorly differentiated (High grade)

T   E.   Geade 4   :   Undifferentiated (High grade)

21. The following are statements regarding classification of benign tumours:

T   A.   A lipoma is a common benign tumor of fat cells

F   B.   A Hamartoma is a benign tumor of cartilage-forming cells

T   C.   Adenomas are benign tumors of gland-forming cells

T   D.   Teratomas contain many cell types such as skin, nerve, brain and thyroid, because they are derived from germ cells

F   E.   A chondroma is a benign tumor that has relatively normal cellular differentiation.

22. The following are statements regarding wound healing:

T   A.   In the inflammatory phase, bacteria and debris are phagocytosed and removed

T   B.   The proliferative phase is characterized by angiogenesis, collagen deposition, granulation tissue formation

T   C.   In angiogenesis, new blood vessels are formed by vascular endothelial cells

F   D.   In maturation and remodeling phase, the wound is made smaller by the action of myofibroblasts

F   E.   In the contraction, collagen is remodeled and realigned along tension lines

23. Systemic factors affecting wound healing include:

T   A.   Inflammation

T   B.   Connective Tissue Disorders

T   C.   Metabolic Diseases

T D. Immunosuppression

F E. Obesity

24. The following are statements regarding primary intention type of wound healing

T A. It involves epidermis and dermis without total penetration of dermis healing by process of epithelialization

T B. When wound edges are brought together so that they are adjacent to each other.

F C. It maximizes scarring

T D. Most surgical wounds heal by primary intention healing

T E. Well-repaired laceration is an example.

25. The following are statements regarding metaplasia

T A. It is an adaptation that replaces one type of epithelium with another

T B. It is accompanied by a loss of endothelial function

T C. The cell of origin for many types of metaplasias are unknown

F D. The metaplastic area should be neglected until revised to normal

T E. Barrett's esophagus is an example

26. The followings are causes of metaplasia:

T A. Cigarette smoke

T B. Bladder stone

T C. Gastro-esophageal reflux

T   D.   Low pH of vagina

F   E.   Sleep deprivation

27.   Major pathological microscopic changes of Dysplasia include:

T   A.   Anisocytosis (cells of unequal size)

T   B.   Poikilocytosis (abnormally shaped cells)

T   C.   Hyperchromatism (excessive pigmentation)

T   D.   Presence of mitotic figures (an unusual number of cells which are currently dividing)

F   E.   Increased nuclear cytopalsmic ratio

28.   The following are statements regarding dysplasia

T   A.   It is the earliest form of pre-cancerous lesion.

F   B.   It is always low grade

T   C.   It generally consists of an expansion of immature cells

T   D.   Dysplasia, in which cell maturation and differentiation are delayed, can be contrasted with metaplasia

T   E.   Myelodysplastic syndrome is an example

29.   The following are statements regarding granuloma

T   A.   It is a medical term for a tiny collection of immune cells known as macrophages

T   B.   The macrophages in granulomas are often referred to as "epithelioid"

T   C.   All granulomas may contain additional cells and matrix, like neutrophils

T   D.   The difference between granulomas and other types of inflammation is that granulomas form in response to antigens that are resistant to "first-responder" inflammatory cells

T   E.   The antigen causing the formation of a granuloma is most often an infectious pathogen.

30. Granulomas are seen in the following diseases:

T   A.   Tuberculosis

T   B.   Histoplasmosis

T   C.   Cat scratch disease

F   D.   Ulcerative collitis

T   E.   Sarcoidosis

31. The following are statements regarding infarction

T   A.   White infarctions affect solid organs such as the spleen.

T   B.   Severe vasoconstriction is a cause of white infarction

F   C.   Red infarctions generally affect the heart

T   D.   Red infarction affects the small intestine

F   E.   White infarction affects loose tissues that allow blood to collect in the infracted zone

32. The following are statements regarding infarction

T   A.   Myocardial infarction is most commonly due to occlusion of a coronary artery.

T   B.   Cerebral infarction can be atherothrombotic or embolic.

T   C.   Splenic infarction can occur asymptomatically.

F   D.   Limb infarction is presented as leg paralysis

T   E.   Eye infarction can cause sudden visual loss.

33.   **The following are statements regarding morphological patterns of necrosis:**

T   A.   Coagulative necrosis is typically seen in hypoxic environments, such as infarction.

T   B.   Liquefactive necrosis is characterized by the digestion of dead cells to form a viscous liquid mass

F   C.   Fibrinoid necrosis shows amorphous granular debris enclosed within a distinctive inflammatory border.

T   D.   Fat necrosis is specialized necrosis of fat tissue

F   E.   Caseous necrosis is usually caused by immune-mediated vascular damage.

34.   **Conditions caused by poor calcium absorption:**

T   A.   Tartar on teeth

F   B.   Hyper spleenism

T   C.   Arthritic bone spurs

T   D.   Kidney stones

T   E.   Gall stones

35. **Infectious agents are known to be carcinogenic include**

T A. Heliobacter pylori : MALT lymphoma

T B. HPV virus : cervical cancer

T C. Hepatitis B virus : liver cancer

T D. EBV virus : a type of lymphoma

T E. Schistosoma haematobium : bladder cancer

36. **The followings are causes of ischemia:**

T A. Atherosclerosis

T B. Hypotention

T C. Sickle cell anemia

F D. Bradycardia

T E. Hypoglycemia

37. **The following are statements regarding malignant tumour:**

T A. There is anaplasia of cells

F B. It resembles cell of origin microcopically

F C. Its growth is slow

T D. There is presence of giant cells.

T E. It metastasizes to distant organs

38. **Benign tumours are characterized by**

T   A.   slow growth

F   B.   absent of capsule

F   C.   metastasis

F   D.   different histological pattern from parent tissue

T   E.   absent of marked necrosis within the tumour

39.   The following are statements regarding chronic inflammation:

T   A.   Tissue destruction is an important feature

T   B.   Fibrosis is a common end result.

F   C.   Granuloma is proliferating blood vessels and fibrous tissue.

T   D.   Granuloma is common in tuberculosis

F   E.   Liquefactive necrosis is found at the centre of granulomas.

40.   The following are statements regarding morphologic patterns of inflammation:

T   A.   Granulomatous inflammation occurs in syphilis.

T   B.   Fibrinous inflammation is commonly seen in serous cavities.

T   C.   Purulent inflammation is characteristically occurs due to infection by pyogenic bacteria such as staphylococci infection.

T   D.   Serous inflammation characterized by the copious effusion of non-viscous serous fluid, commonly produced by mesothelial cells of serous membranes.

T   E.   Ulcerative inflammation occurs near an epithelium can result in the necrotic loss of tissue from the surface.

41. **The following are statements regarding the appearance of granulation tissue:**

T   A.   Light red or dark pink in color, being perfused with new capillary loops or "buds".

T   B.   Soft to the touch

T   C.   Moist

F   D.   Cyst or cavity formation

T   E.   bumpy (granular) in appearance

42. **The following are statements regarding cancer prognosis:**

T   A.   Presence of systemic symptoms has bad prognosis

F   B.   Site of the tumour does not affect prognosis

T   C.   Well differentiated tumours have good prognosis

F   D.   Stage 4 tumours are associated with good prognosis

T   E.   Responsiveness to therapy has good prognosis

43. **Factors that influence development of an infarct include:**

T   A.   Dual blood supply and presence of collaterals.

T   B.   Rate of development of vascular obstruction.

T   C.   Tissue vulnerability to hypoxia

T   D.   Tissue metabolic rate.

F   E.   Hypothyroidism.

44.   The following are statements regarding an infarct

F   A.   Infarcts are classified on the basis of their size.

T   B.   White infarcts occur with arterial occlusion of solid organs

T   C.   Red infarcts occur with venous occlusions in organs with collateral circulation

T   D.   White infarcts can become hemorrhagic with reperfusion.

T   E.   Red infarcts occur in loose tissues.

45.   The following match is true regarding hemorrhage:

T   A.   Chronic blood loss : iron deficiency anemia

T   B.   Thrombocypenia : gum bleeding

T   C.   Car accident with hypovolemia : shock

T   D.   Heamarthrosis :   clotting factor deficiency

F   E.   Hematemesis : presence of blood in sputum

46.   Recognized causes of defective neutrophil function include:

F   A.   Hepatic failure

F   B.   Diabetes inspidus

T   C.   Hodgkins disease

T   D.   Chediak –higashi syndrome

T   E.   Renal failure

47.   Causes of cancer include:

T   A.   Stress

T   B.   Genetics

T   C.   Obesity

T   D.   Infections

T   E.   Both ionizing and non-ionizing radiation.

48.   Effects and complications of shock include:

T   A.   Adult respiratory distress syndrome

T   B.   Acute tubular necrosis

F   C.   Adrenal hyperplasia

T   D.   Disseminated intravascular coagulation

T   E.   Heart failure

49.   The following are statements regarding effects of shock:

T   A.   Heart failure is a complication in hypovolaemic shock

T   B.   Circulatory changes in the lung occur when compensatory mechanisms are failing.

T   C.   Acute ulceration of the stomach and duodenum may complicate shock.

F   D.   The secretory function of the kidneys is sometimes disturbed in shock

T   E.   Adrenal haemorrhage occurs occasionally in severe shock.

50. **The following are statements regarding shock:**

T   A.   Cardiogenic shock results from myocardial pump failure caused by intrinsic myocardial damage.

T   B.   Hypovolemic shock is associated with fractures of bones

F   C.   Anaphylactic shock initiated by a generalized IgA mediated response.

T   D.   Cyanotic skin is clinical presentation in cardiogenic shock.

T   E.   Old age is a factor favoring progression of shock

1.2 General Microbiology

1.2.a Questions without answers

1.   Differences between Gram-negative and Gram-positive cell walls include:

A.   Gram-negative cell wall has a thicker layer of peptidoglycan.

B.   Gram-positive cell wall contains lipoproteins which stabilize the outer membrane.

C.   Periplasmic space containing detoxifying enzymes is only found in a Gram-positive cell wall.

D.   Lipid A is the toxic component of an endotoxin released upon lysis of a Gram-negative cell wall.

E.   Considerable amounts of teichoic and teichuronic acids are found in Gram-positive cell walls.

2.   Bacterial spores

A.   are usually found in Gram-negative bacteria.

B.   can remain metabolically inert for years.

C.   contain high concentration of calcium dipicolinate.

D.   are structures of reproduction.

E.   are used in the evaluation of the sterilization efficacy in autoclaves.

3. **The following are statements regarding bacterial pathogenicity:**

   A.   Biofilm formation contributes to pathogenicity of *Staphylococcus epidermidis*.

   B.   Endotoxins released by Gram-negative bacteria can be converted to toxoid.

   C.   Encapsulated bacteria exhibit anti-phagocytic property.

   D.   Coagulase produced by *Staphylococcus aureus* allows its easy spread through tissues.

   E.   The pili of *Neisseria gonorrhoeae* mediate its attachment to the urinary tract epithelium.

4. **Exotoxins**

   A.   are excreted by living cells with high concentration in liquid medium.

   B.   cannot be converted to toxoids.

   C.   do not bind to specific receptors on cells.

   D.   produce fever in the host due to the release of interleukin-1 and other mediators.

   E.   are synthesized under the control of extra-chromosomal genes.

5. **The following are statements regarding genetic transfer:**

   A.   Transduction is a process of uptake of fragments of naked DNA.

   B.   Transformation is a process of the DNA transfer via

bacteriophage.

C. Double-stranded DNA is transferred during conjugation.

D. In conjugation, the DNA is passed directly by cell-to-cell contact via the sex pilus.

E. Transduction is termed as specialized if the selection of the transferred genes is at random.

6. **Plasmids**

A. are extra-chromosomal genetic material.

B. are incapable of autonomous replication.

C. carry genes which code for only one antibiotic resistance at any one time.

D. are only found in Gram-negative bacteria.

E. mediate toxin production.

7. **The following are statements regarding sterilization/ disinfection:**

A. Boiling at 100°C kills all vegetative cells including spores.

B. Autoclave uses steam under pressure to reach optimum temperature of 121°C.

C. Ethylene oxide is used for sterilization of endoscopes.

D. Pasteurization is the process which eliminates spores in milk.

E. Filtration is the preferred method of sterilizing heat-sensitive solution.

8. **Antiseptics**

    A.   are used to reduce the number of microorganisms without causing tissue toxicity.

    B.   are used in pre-operative skin preparation.

    C.   include 70% alcohol.

    D.   have activity against bacterial spores.

    E.   demonstrate enhanced activity in the presence of pus.

9. *Staphylococcus epidermidis*

    A.   is a normal flora of the skin.

    B.   appears as beta-hemolytic colonies on blood agar.

    C.   is catalase negative and coagulase positive.

    D.   produces extracellular slime.

    E.   is an important cause of prosthetic valve endocarditis.

10.

The following are the differences and similarities in the characteristics of Viridans *Streptococcus* and *Streptococcus pneumoniae*:

	Viridans *Streptococcus*		*Streptococcus pneumoniae*
A.	Gram-positive diplococcus	:	Gram-positive coccus in clusters
B.	Gamma-hemolytic colonies	:	Beta-hemolytic colonies

C.	Sensitive to optochin	:	Resistant to optochin
D.	Insoluble in bile	:	Soluble in bile
E.	Normal flora of upper respiratory tract	:	Normal flora of upper respiratory tract

11. *Enterococcus* **sp.**

    A.   is a Gram-positive coccus typically arranged in pairs or short chains.

    B.   has Lancefield group C antigen.

    C.   is part of the normal flora of the human gastrointestinal tract.

    D.   is one of causative agents of nosocomial infections.

    E.   is usually sensitive to cephalosporins.

12. **The following are statements regarding Family**
Enterobactericaeae:

    A.   The family includes several genera which are oxidase positive.

    B.   Majority of the members are Gram-negative facultative anaerobes.

    C.   They can either be lactose fermenters or non-lactose fermenters on MacConkey agar.

    D.   All members of the family are normal flora of the gastrointestinal tract

E.   They are identified based on carbohydrate fermentation reactions.

13.   *Haemophilus influenzae*

A.   is a normal flora of the upper respiratory tract.

B.   requires only factor X for growth.

C.   shows satellite phenomenon around the colonies of staphylococci.

D.   serotype f causes most of the severe infections.

E.   is a common causative agent of acute epiglotitis.

14.   *Escherichia coli*

A.   appears non-lactose fermenting colonies on MacConkey agar.

B.   is a commensal of the gastrointestinal tract.

C.   of the enteropathogenic type produces shiga-like toxin.

D.   is one of the causative agents of neonatal meningitis.

E.   is innately resistant to quinolones.

15.   *Klebsiella* **sp.**

A.   is a non-motile Gram-negative bacillus

B.   appears as mucoid colonies on MacConkey agar.

C.   is one of the causative agents of urinary tract infection.

D.   is found as commensals in the gastrointestinal tract.

E.   is not known to produce extended-spectrum beta-lactamase (
      ESBL).

16.   *Neisseria meningitidis* and *Neisseria gonorrhoeae* share
      the following characteristics. These organisms

A.   are intracellular Gram-negative diplococci.

B.   have pili.

C.   have outer membrane protein.

D.   both ferment glucose and maltose.

E.   are encapsulated.

17.   *Campylobacter* sp.

A.   is a seagull-shaped Gram-negative organism.

B.   is acquired via ingestion of contaminated food or milk.

C.   is associated with MALT lymphoma.

D.   can be detected in biopsy by rapid urease test.

E.   is sensitive to erythromycin.

18.   *Actinomyces* sp

A.   is an anaerobic Gram-positive bacillus in filaments.

B.   is weakly acid-fast.

C.   is usually found as normal flora of the oral cavity.

D.   colonizes intrauterine contraceptive devices.

E.   is sensitive to trimethoprim-sulphamethoxazole.

19.   **The following are pairs regarding *Chlamydia* spp. and their associated infections:**

A.   *Chlamydia trachomatis (D-K)*   :   inclusion conjunctivitis

B.   *Chlamydia pneumoniae*   :   atypical pneumonia

C.   *Chlamydia trachomatis (L$_1$-L$_3$)*   :   trachoma

D.   *Chlamydia psittaci*   :   ornithosis

E.   *Chlamydia trachomatis (A,B,C)*   :   non-gonococcal urethritis

20.   *Mycoplasma* **spp.**

A.   have Gram-positive cell wall.

B.   appear as small colonies with fried egg appearance.

C.   possess adhesion protein P1 which acts as a superantigen.

D.   have an affinity for mammalian cell membranes.

E.   are resistant to erythromycin.

21.   *Ureaplasma urealyticum.*

A.   requires urea for growth.

B.   is the most common cause of non-gonococcal urethritis in men.

C.   is commonly found in the female genital tract.

D.   is associated with lung disease in premature low birth weight infants.

E.   is sensitive to tetracycline.

22.   **The following are statements regarding *Coxiella burnetii*:**

A.   Ticks are an important vector in human disease.

B.   It can undergo antigenic variation.

C.   It is one of the causes of culture-negative infective endocarditis.

D.   Rash is the most common clinical manifestation of its infection.

E.   High titer of antibody to phase I antigen is detected in acute infection.

23.   *Orientia tsutsugamushi*

A.   is the causative agent of Brill-Zinsser disease.

B.   is transmitted by tick bites.

C.   can be easily isolated from blood cultures.

D.   produces eschar at the site of its entry into the body.

E.   is sensitive to doxycycline.

24. *Rickettsia* **sp**

    A.   is an obligate intracellular organism.

    B.   is best detected in infected cells by Gram stain.

    C.   is transmitted via bites of infected arthropod.

    D.   causes vasculitis as the primary pathological lesion.

    E.   can be easily cultured from clinical specimens.

25. *Mycobacterium tuberculosis*

    A.   is an acid-fast bacillus.

    B.   stimulates predominantly a humoral-mediated immune response.

    C.   requires 4-6 weeks to grow on Lowenstein-Jensen medium.

    D.   causes typical caseation necrosis.

    E.   is easily be killed by alveolar macrophages.

26. **The following are statements regarding spirochetes:**

    A.   *Borrelia burgdorferi* is the causative organism of relapsing fevers.

    B.   *Leptospira interrogans* are shed in large numbers in urine of rats.

    C.   *Borrelia recurrentis* undergoes antigenic variation.

    D.   Treponema pallidum can be easily isolated from blood cultures

    E.   The microhemagglutination assay for *Treponema pallidum* (MHA-TP) becomes negative after pencillin therapy.

27. **Lyme disease**

    A. is caused by *Borrelia burgdorferi*.

    B. Presents with erythema migrans, a skin lesion with central clearing.

    C. is transmitted via bites of mosquitoes.

    D. occurs in stages with early and late manifestations

    E. is treated with doxycycline

28. **A positive VDRL (Venereal Disease Research Laboratory) test with negative TPHA (*Treponema pallidum* hemagglutination) and FTA (fluorescent treponemal antibody) tests is consistent with the following conditions:**

    A. yaws.

    B. Primary syphilis

    C. Secondary syphilis

    D. malaria

    E. systemic lupus erythematosus

29. **The following laboratory techniques help in diagnosis of bacterial infections:**

    A. microscopic examination of Gram-stained smears of clinical specimens.

    B. culture and identification of the causative bacteria.

C.   fatty acid analysis of anaerobes by gas liquid chromatography.

D.   detection of two-fold rise in antibody titers between the acute and convalescent sera.

E.   nucleic acid probes for detection of organisms which are difficult to grow.

30. **The following are statements regarding the characteristics of fungi:**

A.   Dematiaceous fungi are characterised by the presence of melanin in their cell walls.

B.   Vegetative hyphae project above the colony and bear the reproductive structures.

C.   Most fungi grow on Sabouraud's dextrose agar.

D.   Arthroconidia are spores resulting from fragmentation of hyphae.

E.   Fungi which are capable of sexual reproduction are classified as imperfect fungi.

31. **Dimorphic fungi**

A.   are characterized by the presence of pigments in the cell walls.

B.   develop into filamentous form when incubated at 37°C.

C.   develop into oval yeast cells when incubated at 30°C.

D.   present as yeasts within the macrophages in tissues.

E.   causes pulmonary infection via inhalation of spores.

32. *Candida albicans*

    A.   is an encapsulated yeast.

    B.   reproduces by fragmentation of the pseudohyphae.

    C.   causes esophagitis in patients with AIDS.

    D.   is a normal flora of the genital tract.

    E.   is sensitive to fluconazole.

33. *Cryptococcus neoformans*

    A.   is a Gram-positive yeast with budding.

    B.   can be detected by India ink preparation.

    C.   does not grow on Sabouraud's dextrose agar.

    D.   can be isolated from pigeon droppings.

    E.   is one of the causative agents of meningitis.

34. **A 10-year-old boy complained of "itching rash" on his forearm. On examination, red, circular with vesiculated border and a healing central area is seen. The following statements are regarding the likely causative organism:**

    A.   It is likely to be one of the dermatophytes.

    B.   The morphology of the macroconidia and microconidia helps in the identification.

    C.   Its infections are usually confined to the skin.

    D.   It can only be detected in skin scraping obtained from centre of the skin lesion.

E.   Amphotericin B is the antifungal agent of choice.

35.

Aspergillosis

A.

is caused by a dimorphic fungus.

B.

presents with a fungal ball in a pre-existing lung cavity.

C.

is a fatal disease in bone marrow transplant patients.

D.

causes allergic bronchopulmonary disease.

E.

is treated with amphotericin B.

36.   The following are pairs regarding fungi and their characteristic features:

A.	*Candida albicans*	:	Encapsulated budding yeast seen in India ink preparation of cerebrospinal fluid.
B.	*Sporothrix schenckii*	:	A mold that form fungal ball in the pre-existing tuberculous cavity.
C.	*Aspergillus sp*	:	A dimorphic mold that typically transmitted via trauma to the skin.
D.	*Cryptococcus neoformans*	:	A budding yeast that is a member of the normal vaginal flora.
E.	*Penicillium marneffei*	:	Its presence in blood is one of the AIDS-defining illnesses.

37.   Viruses

A.   are obligate intracellular parasites.

B.   consist of nucleic acid genomes packaged into protein coats.

C.   can be released from the cells by budding from the plasma membrane.

D.   of Picornaviridae family attach to host cells via hemagglutinin spikes.

E.   with negative-sense RNA can act as mRNA directly.

38.   Steps in the replication of enveloped DNA viruses include

A.   Uncoating to release the nucleic acids.

B.   Transcription of early and late mRNA.

C.   Synthesis of structural proteins.

D.   Assembly in the cytoplasm.

E.   Release by sudden rupture of infected cells.

39.   Outcome of viral infections includes

A.   Inapparent infection occurs when the infected tissue is undamaged.

B.   Majority of acute infections recover with residual effects.

C.   Latent infection is when the infecting virus resides in certain tissues for life.

D.   Development of disease occurs only after a long incubation period.

E.   Progression to tumors is often associated with permissive type of infections

40.   The following are statements regarding latent viral infection:

A.   It is a form of persistent infection.

B.   It occurs when the nucleic acid integrates itself into the host DNA as a provirus.

C.   The infectious virus is usually undetectable.

D.   Chickenpox is a typical example.

E.   Trigeminal ganglion is the site of latency of cytomegalovirus.

41.   Influenza virus

A.   has a single-stranded, positive-sense RNA genome.

B.   frequently establishes persistent infections in the lung.

C.   is strictly a human pathogen.

D.   has envelope which contains hemagglutinin and neuramidase.

E.   undergoes genetic reassortment among members of the same genus.

42.   Mumps virus

A.   is a DNA virus with several serological types.

B.   has predilection for glandular tissues.

C.   is transmitted by inhalation of infected respiratory secretions.

D. is one of the causative agents of aseptic meningitis.

E. does not induce long-lasting immunity.

43. Respiratory syncytial virus

A   belongs to the family Orthomyxoviridae.

B. causes acute laryngotracheobronchitis (Croup) in infants under 1 year of age.

C. does not grow in cell culture.

D. is found in high titers in respiratory tract secretions.

E. frequently causes latent infections.

44. Coxsackie A virus

A. has a single-stranded RNA genome.

B. replicates in the gastrointestinal tract.

C. causes pleurodynia (also known as epidemic myalgia).

D. does not show any cytopathic effects in cell culture.

E. is the main agent of viral gastroenteritis in adults.

45. Epstein-Barr virus

A. is a DNA virus.

B. remains latent in B lymphocytes following primary infection.

C. causes heterophile-negative infectious mononucleosis.

D. does not possess any oncogenic properties.

E. can be transmitted via contact with saliva.

46. Herpes simplex virus type 2

A. is a double-stranded DNA virus.

B. remains latent in the trigeminal ganglion.

C. is spread by direct contact with infected saliva.

D. causes severe keratoconjunctivitis.

E. is sensitive to acyclovir.

47. Cytomegalovirus

A. belongs to the herpesvirus family.

B. does not cause latent infections.

C. produces a characteristic cytopathic effect with perinuclear cytoplasmic inclusion.

D. causes heterophile-positive infectious mononucleosis.

E. is sensitive to ganciclovir.

48. Human papillomavirus

A. is a double-stranded DNA virus.

B. causes infections at the cutaneous and mucosal sites.

C. causes genital warts known as condylomata lata.

D.   can be transmitted via direct contact.

E.   of serotypes 6 and 8 are associated with cervical carcinoma.

49.   Adenovirus

A.   is a RNA virus.

B.   of types 40 and 41 are the major cause gastroenteritis in adults.

C.   persists for long periods in the adenoids.

D.   is associated with epidemic keratoconjunctivitis.

E.   is spread via respiratory secretions.

50.   The following are pairs regarding oncogenic viruses and their associated tumors:

A.   Epstein-Barr virus   :   Burkitt's lymphoma

B.   Human papillomavirus   :   Cervical cancer

C.   Hepatitis A virus   :   Hepatocellular carcinoma

D.   Herpes simplex type 2   :   Cervical cancer

E.   HIV-1   :   T cell leukemia

1.2 General Microbiology

1.2.b Questions with answers

1. Differences between Gram-negative and Gram-positive cell walls include:

F A. Gram-negative cell wall has a thicker layer of peptidoglycan.

F B. Gram-positive cell wall contains lipoproteins which stabilize the outer membrane.

F C. Periplasmic space containing detoxifying enzymes is only found in a Gram-positive cell wall.

T D. Lipid A is the toxic component of an endotoxin released upon lysis of a Gram-negative cell wall.

T E. Considerable amounts of teichoic and teichuronic acids are found in Gram-positive cell walls.

2. Bacterial spores

F A. are usually found in Gram-negative bacteria.

T B. can remain metabolically inert for years.

T C. contain high concentration of calcium dipicolinate.

F D. are structures of reproduction.

T   E.   are used in the evaluation of the sterilization efficacy in autoclaves.

3. The following are statements regarding bacterial pathogenicity:

T   A.   Biofilm formation contributes to pathogenicity of *Staphylococcus epidermidis*.

F   B.   Endotoxins released by Gram-negative bacteria can be converted to toxoid.

T   C.   Encapsulated bacteria exhibit anti-phagocytic property.

F   D.   Coagulase produced by *Staphylococcus aureus* allows its easy spread through tissues.

T   E.   The pili of *Neisseria gonorrhoeae* mediate its attachment to the urinary tract epithelium.

4. Exotoxins

T   A.   are excreted by living cells with high concentration in liquid medium.

F   B.   cannot be converted to toxoids.

F   C.   do not bind to specific receptors on cells.

F   D.   produce fever in the host due to the release of interleukin-1 and other mediators.

T   E.   are synthesized under the control of extra-chromosomal genes.

5. The following are statements regarding genetic transfer:

F   A.   Transduction is a process of uptake of fragments of naked

DNA.

F   B.   Transformation is a process of the DNA transfer via bacteriophage.

F   C.   Double-stranded DNA is transferred during conjugation.

T   D.   In conjugation, the DNA is passed directly by cell-to-cell contact via the sex pilus.

F   E.   Transduction is termed as specialized if the selection of the transferred genes is at random.

6.   Plasmids

T   A.   are extra-chromosomal genetic material.

F   B.   are incapable of autonomous replication.

F   C.   carry genes which code for only one antibiotic resistance at any one time.

F   D.   are only found in Gram-negative bacteria.

T   E.   mediate toxin production.

7.   The following are statements regarding sterilization/ disinfection:

F   A.   Boiling at 100°C kills all vegetative cells including spores.

T   B.   Autoclave uses steam under pressure to reach optimum temperature of 121°C.

T   C.   Ethylene oxide is used for sterilization of endoscopes.

F   D.   Pasteurization is the process which eliminates spores in milk.

T   E.   Filtration is the preferred method of sterilizing heat-sensitive solution.

8. Antiseptics

T   A.   are used to reduce the number of microorganisms without causing tissue toxicity.

T   B.   are used in pre-operative skin preparation.

T   C.   include 70% alcohol.

F   D.   have activity against bacterial spores.

F   E.   demonstrate enhanced activity in the presence of pus.

9. *Staphylococcus epidermidis*

T   A.   is a normal flora of the skin.

F   B.   appears as beta-hemolytic colonies on blood agar.

F   C.   is catalase negative and coagulase positive.

T   D.   produces extracellular slime.

T   E.   is an important cause of prosthetic valve endocarditis.

10.

The following are the differences and similarities in the characteristics of Viridans *Streptococcus* and *Streptococcus pneumoniae*:

	Viridans *Streptococcus*		*Streptococcus pneumoniae*
F			
A.	Gram-positive diplococcus	:	Gram-positive coccus

59

in clusters

F

B.	Gamma-hemolytic colonies	:	Beta-hemolytic colonies

F

C.	Sensitive to optochin	:	Resistant to optochin

T

D.	Insoluble in bile	:	Soluble in bile

T

E.	Normal flora of upper respiratory tract	:	Normal flora of upper respiratory tract

11. *Enterococcus* sp.

T   A. is a Gram-positive coccus typically arranged in pairs or short chains.

F   B. has Lancefield group C antigen.

T   C. is part of the normal flora of the human gastrointestinal tract.

T   D. is one of causative agents of nosocomial infections.

F   E. is usually sensitive to cephalosporins.

12. The following are statements regarding Family *Enterobactericaeae:*

F   A. The family includes several genera which are oxidase positive.

T   B. Majority of the members are Gram-negative facultative anaerobes.

T   C. They can either be lactose fermenters or non-lactose

fermenters on MacConkey agar.

F   D.   All members of the family are normal flora of the
         gastrointestinal tract

T   E.   They are identified based on carbohydrate fermentation
         reactions.

13. *Haemophilus influenzae*

T   A.   is a normal flora of the upper respiratory tract.

F   B.   requires only factor X for growth.

T   C.   shows satellite phenomenon around the colonies of
         staphylococci.

F   D.   serotype f causes most of the severe infections.

T   E.   is a common causative agent of acute epiglotitis.

14. *Escherichia coli*

F   A.   appears non-lactose fermenting colonies on MacConkey agar.

T   B.   is a commensal of the gastrointestinal tract.

F   C.   of the enteropathogenic type produces shiga-like toxin.

T   D.   is one of the causative agents of neonatal meningitis.

F   E.   is innately resistant to quinolones.

15. *Klebsiella* sp.

T   A.   is a non-motile Gram-negative bacillus

T   B.   appears as mucoid colonies on MacConkey agar.

T   C.   is one of the causative agents of urinary tract infection.

T   D.   is found as commensals in the gastrointestinal tract.

F   E.   is not known to produce extended-spectrum beta-lactamase (ESBL).

16.   *Neisseria meningitidis* and *Neisseria gonorrhoeae* share the following characteristics. These organisms

T   A.   are intracellular Gram-negative diplococci.

T   B.   have pili.

T   C.   have outer membrane protein.

F   D.   both ferment glucose and maltose.

F   E.   are encapsulated.

17.   *Campylobacter* sp.

T   A.   is a seagull-shaped Gram-negative organism.

T   B.   is acquired via ingestion of contaminated food or milk.

F   C.   is associated with MALT lymphoma.

F   D.   can be detected in biopsy by rapid urease test.

T   E.   is sensitive to erythromycin.

18.   *Actinomyces* sp

T   A.   is an anaerobic Gram-positive bacillus in filaments.

F   B.   is weakly acid-fast.

T   C.   is usually found as normal flora of the oral cavity.

T   D.   colonizes intrauterine contraceptive devices.

F   E.   is sensitive to trimethoprim-sulphamethoxazole.

19.   **The following are pairs regarding *Chlamydia* spp. and their associated infections:**

T   A.   *Chlamydia trachomatis (D-K)*   :   inclusion conjunctivitis

T   B.   *Chlamydia pneumoniae*   :   atypical pneumonia

F   C.   *Chlamydia trachomatis (L$_1$-L$_3$)*   :   trachoma

T   D.   *Chlamydia psittaci*   :   ornithosis

F   E.   *Chlamydia trachomatis (A,B,C)*   :   non-gonococcal urethritis

20.   ***Mycoplasma* spp.**

F   A.   have Gram-positive cell wall.

T   B.   appear as small colonies with fried egg appearance.

T   C.   possess adhesion protein P1 which acts as a superantigen.

T   D.   have an affinity for mammalian cell membranes.

F   E.   are resistant to erythromycin.

21. *Ureaplasma urealyticum.*

T   A.   requires urea for growth.

F   B.   is the most common cause of non-gonococcal urethritis in men.

T   C.   is commonly found in the female genital tract.

T   D.   is associated with lung disease in premature low birth weight infants.

F   E.   is sensitive to tetracycline.

22. **The following are statements regarding *Coxiella burnetii*:**

F   A.   Ticks are an important vector in human disease.

T   B.   It can undergo antigenic variation.

T   C.   It is one of the causes of culture-negative infective endocarditis.

F   D.   Rash is the most common clinical manifestation of its infection.

F   E.   High titer of antibody to phase I antigen is detected in acute infection.

23. *Orientia tsutsugamushi*

F   A.   is the causative agent of Brill-Zinsser disease.

F   B.   is transmitted by tick bites.

F   C.   can be easily isolated from blood cultures.

T   D.   produces eschar at the site of its entry into the body.

T   E.   is sensitive to doxycycline.

24.   *Rickettsia* sp

T   A.   is an obligate intracellular organism.

F   B.   is best detected in infected cells by Gram stain.

T   C.   is transmitted via bites of infected arthropod.

T   D.   causes vasculitis as the primary pathological lesion.

F   E.   can be easily cultured from clinical specimens.

25.   *Mycobacterium tuberculosis*

T   A.   is an acid-fast bacillus.

F   B.   stimulates predominantly a humoral-mediated immune response.

T   C.   requires 4-6 weeks to grow on Lowenstein-Jensen medium.

T   D.   causes typical caseation necrosis.

F   E.   is easily be killed by alveolar macrophages.

26.   The following are statements regarding spirochetes:

F   A.   *Borrelia burgdorferi* is the causative organism of relapsing fevers.

T   B.   *Leptospira interrogans* are shed in large numbers in urine of rats.

T   C.   *Borrelia recurrentis* undergoes antigenic variation.

F   D.   Treponema pallidum can be easily isolated from blood cultures

F   E.   The microhemagglutination assay for *Treponema pallidum* (MHA-TP) becomes negative after pencillin therapy.

27.   Lyme disease

T   A.   is caused by *Borrelia burgdorferi.*

T   B.   Presents with erythema migrans, a skin lesion with central clearing.

F   C.   is transmitted via bites of mosquitoes.

T   D.   occurs in stages with early and late manifestations

F   E.   is treated with doxycycline

28.   A positive VDRL (Venereal Disease Research Laboratory) test with negative TPHA (*Treponema pallidum* hemagglutination) and FTA (fluorescent treponemal antibody) tests is consistent with the following conditions:

F   A.   yaws.

F   B.   Primary syphilis

F   C.   Secondary syphilis

T   D.   malaria

T   E.   systemic lupus erythematosus

29.   The following laboratory techniques help in diagnosis of bacterial infections:

T   A.   microscopic examination of Gram-stained smears of clinical specimens.

T   B.   culture and identification of the causative bacteria.

T   C.   fatty acid analysis of anaerobes by gas liquid chromatography.

F   D.   detection of two-fold rise in antibody titers between the acute and convalescent sera.

T   E.   nucleic acid probes for detection of organisms which are difficult to grow.

30. The following are statements regarding the characteristics of fungi:

T   A.   Dematiaceous fungi are characterised by the presence of melanin in their cell walls.

F   B.   Vegetative hyphae project above the colony and bear the reproductive structures.

T   C.   Most fungi grow on Sabouraud's dextrose agar.

T   D.   Arthroconidia are spores resulting from fragmentation of hyphae.

F   E.   Fungi which are capable of sexual reproduction are classified as imperfect fungi.

31. Dimorphic fungi

F   A.   are characterized by the presence of pigments in the cell walls.

F   B.   develop into filamentous form when incubated at 37°C.

F   C.   develop into oval yeast cells when incubated at 30°C.

T   D.   present as yeasts within the macrophages in tissues.

T   E.   causes pulmonary infection via inhalation of spores.

32. *Candida albicans*

F   A.   is an encapsulated yeast.

F   B.   reproduces by fragmentation of the pseudohyphae.

T   C.   causes esophagitis in patients with AIDS.

T   D.   is a normal flora of the genital tract.

T   E.   is sensitive to fluconazole.

33. *Cryptococcus neoformans*

T   A.   is a Gram-positive yeast with budding.

T   B.   can be detected by India ink preparation.

F   C.   does not grow on Sabouraud's dextrose agar.

T   D.   can be isolated from pigeon droppings.

T   E.   is one of the causative agents of meningitis.

34. A 10-year-old boy complained of "itching rash" on his forearm. On examination, red, circular with vesiculated border and a healing central area is seen. The following statements are regarding the likely causative organism:

T   A.   It is likely to be one of the dermatophytes.

T   B.   The morphology of the macroconidia and microconidia helps in the identification.

F   C.   Its infections are usually confined to the skin.

F   D.   It can only be detected in skin scraping obtained from centre of the skin lesion.

T . E.   Amphotericin B is the antifungal agent of choice.

35.

Aspergillosis

F   A.
    is caused by a dimorphic fungus.

T   B.
    presents with a fungal ball in a pre-existing lung cavity.

T   C.
    is a fatal disease in bone marrow transplant patients.

T   D.
    causes allergic bronchopulmonary disease.

T   E.
    is treated with amphotericin B.

36. The following are pairs regarding fungi and their characteristic features:

F   A.   *Candida albicans*   :   Encapsulated budding yeast seen in India ink preparation of cerebrospinal fluid.

F   B.   *Sporothrix schenckii*   :   A mold that form fungal ball in the pre-existing tuberculous cavity.

F   C.   *Aspergillus sp*   :   A dimorphic mold that typically transmitted via trauma to the skin.

F   D.   *Cryptococcus*   :   A budding yeast that is a member *neoformans*   of the normal vaginal flora.

T   E.   *Penicillium marneffei*   :   Its presence in blood is one of the AIDS-defining illnesses.

37.   Viruses

T   A.   are obligate intracellular parasites.

T   B.   consist of nucleic acid genomes packaged into protein coats.

T   C.   can be released from the cells by budding from the plasma membrane.

F   D.   of Picornaviridae family attach to host cells via hemagglutinin spikes.

F   E.   with negative-sense RNA can act as mRNA directly.

38.   Steps in the replication of enveloped DNA viruses include

T   A.   Uncoating to release the nucleic acids.

T   B.   Transcription of early and late mRNA.

T   C.   Synthesis of structural proteins.

F   D.   Assembly in the cytoplasm.

F   E.   Release by sudden rupture of infected cells.

39.   Outcome of viral infections includes

T   A.   Inapparent infection occurs when the infected tissue is undamaged.

F   B.   Majority of acute infections recover with residual effects.

T   C.   Latent infection is when the infecting virus resides in certain tissues for life.

T   D.   Development of disease occurs only after a long incubation period.

F   E.   Progression to tumors is often associated with permissive type of infections

40.   The following are statements regarding latent viral infection:

T   A.   It is a form of persistent infection.

T   B.   It occurs when the nucleic acid integrates itself into the host DNA as a provirus.

T   C.   The infectious virus is usually undetectable.

F   D.   Chickenpox is a typical example.

F   E.   Trigeminal ganglion is the site of latency of cytomegalovirus.

41.   Influenza virus

F   A.   has a single-stranded, positive-sense RNA genome.

F   B.   frequently establishes persistent infections in the lung.

F   C.   is strictly a human pathogen.

T   D.   has envelope which contains hemagglutinin and neuramidase.

T   E.   undergoes genetic reassortment among members of the same genus.

42. Mumps virus

F   A.   is a DNA virus with several serological types.

T   B.   has predilection for glandular tissues.

T   C.   is transmitted by inhalation of infected respiratory secretions.

T   D.   is one of the causative agents of aseptic meningitis.

F   E.   does not induce long-lasting immunity.

43. Respiratory syncytial virus

F   A   belongs to the family Orthomyxoviridae.

T   B.   causes acute laryngotracheobronchitis (Croup) in infants under 1 year of age.

F   C.   does not grow in cell culture.

T   D.   is found in high titers in respiratory tract secretions.

F   E.   frequently causes latent infections.

44. Coxsackie A virus

T   A.   has a single-stranded RNA genome.

T   B.   replicates in the gastrointestinal tract.

F   C.   causes pleurodynia (also known as epidemic myalgia).

F   D.   does not show any cytopathic effects in cell culture.

F   E.   is the main agent of viral gastroenteritis in adults.

45. Epstein-Barr virus

T   A.   is a DNA virus.

T   B.   remains latent in B lymphocytes following primary infection.

F   C.   causes heterophile-negative infectious mononucleosis.

F   D.   does not possess any oncogenic properties.

T   E.   can be transmitted via contact with saliva.

46. Herpes simplex virus type 2

T   A.   is a double-stranded DNA virus.

F   B.   remains latent in the trigeminal ganglion.

F   C.   is spread by direct contact with infected saliva.

F   D.   causes severe keratoconjunctivitis.

T   E.   is sensitive to acyclovir.

47. Cytomegalovirus

T   A.   belongs to the herpesvirus family.

F   B.   does not cause latent infections.

T   C.   produces a characteristic cytopathic effect with perinuclear cytoplasmic inclusion.

F   D.   causes heterophile-positive infectious mononucleosis.

T   E.   is sensitive to ganciclovir.

48. Human papillomavirus

T   A.   is a double-stranded DNA virus.

T   B.   causes infections at the cutaneous and mucosal sites.

F   C.   causes genital warts known as condylomata lata.

T   D.   can be transmitted via direct contact.

F   E.   of serotypes 6 and 8 are associated with cervical carcinoma.

49. Adenovirus

F   A.   is a RNA virus.

F   B.   of types 40 and 41 are the major cause gastroenteritis in adults.

T   C.   persists for long periods in the adenoids.

T   D.   is associated with epidemic keratoconjunctivitis.

T   E.   is spread via respiratory secretions.

50. The following are pairs regarding oncogenic viruses and their associated tumors:

T   A.   Epstein-Barr virus   :   Burkitt's lymphoma

T   B.   Human papillomavirus   :   Cervical cancer

F   C.   Hepatitis A virus   :   Hepatocellular carcinoma

T   D.   Herpes simplex type 2   :   Cervical cancer

F   E.   HIV-1   :   T cell leukemia

2 CARDIOVASCULAR SYSTEM

2.1 Pathology of Cardiovascular System

2.1.a Questions without answers

1.   The following are statements regarding aortic dissection:

A.   It may or may not be associated with marked dilatation of the aorta.

B.   It can be iatrogenic.

C.   It can extend along the aorta toward the heart.

D.   In most cases, there is specific underlying preexisting and causal pathology is seen in the aortic wall.

E.   Hypertension is clearly the major risk factor overall.

2.   The following are statements regarding aortic dissection:

A.   Some dissections are related to the inherited connective tissue disorders.

B.   The cause of spontaneous dissections not associated with hypertension is unknown.

C.   The classic clinical symptoms are the gradual onset of excruciating pain.

D.   The most common cause of death is rupture of the dissection.

E.   Myocardial infarction is not common clinical manifestations.

3.   The following are statements regarding rheumatic fever:

A.   It follows a Group B beta-hemolytic streptococcal infection.

B.   The body produces antibodies that cross react with human tissues.

C.   The characteristic lesion of acute rheumatic fever is the Aschoff body

D.   The aortic valve is the most affected valve.

E.   When pericarditis is present, it rarely affects cardiac function.

4.   The following are statements regarding rheumatic fever:

A.   It is acute immunologically mediated.

B.   It is multisystem inflammatory disease.

C.   It follows an episode of group A srteptococcal pharingitis.

D.   It often follows streptococcal infection of skin.

E.   It causes chronic deformity of the large joints.

5.   Predisposing factors of cardiac failure include:

A. Coronary blood supply insufficiency.

B. Systemic hypertension.

C. Thyrotoxicosis.

D. Pneumonitis.

E. Diabetes mellitus.

6. **Symptoms of heart failure include:**

   A. Dyspnea

   B. Persistent cough

   C. Blood tinged sputum

   D. Diarrhoea

   E. Edema in feet

7. **The following are statements regarding Aschoff bodies:**

   A. They are nodules found in the hearts of individuals with chronic heart disease.

   B. Fully developed Aschoff bodies are granulomatous structures consisting of fibrinoid change.

   C. They contain lymphocytic infiltration.

   D. There are abnormal macrophages surrounding necrotic centers

   E. The Aschoff nodules are spheroidal or fusiform distinct tiny structures.

8.   **Major risk factors of angina pectoris include:**

  A.   Age ($\geq$ 55 years for men, $\geq$ 65 for women)

  B.   Cigarette smoking

  C.   Diabetes mellitus

  D.   Dyslipidemia

  E.   Hypertension

9.   **The following are statements regarding infective endocarditis:**

  A.   Gram negative bacilli infect the valves in drug abusers.

  B.   Prosthetic valves are associated with a lower risk of developing infective endocarditis.

  C.   Glomerulonephritis is a complication.

  D.   Vegetations are large and bulky.

  E.   Vegetations may extend to the chordate tendinae.

10.   **The following are statements regarding pulmonary vascular diseases:**

  A.   Heart failure cells are seen in pulmonary thromboembolism

  B.   Pulmonary venous hypertension is caused by congestive heart failure.

  C.   Adult respiratory distress syndrome can be a complication of sepsis.

  D.   Cor pulmonale is acute left heart failure due to systemic hypertension.

E. Recurrent thromboemboli in the lungs lead to pulmonary hypertension

11. **The following are statements regarding atherosclerosis:**

A. It is a chronic disease that remains asymptomatic for decades

B. Atherosclerotic plaques are rich in extracellular matrix and smooth muscle cells.

C. Unstable plaques are rich in macrophages and foam cells

D. Atherosclerosis affects the entire artery tree

E. Diabetes is a risk factor

12. **Risk factors of atherosclerosis include:**

A. High serum concentration of low-density lipoprotein

B. High serum concentration of functioning high density lipoprotein

C. Smoking

D. Hypertension

E. Vitamin B_6 deficiency

13. **Ischemic heart disease presents with any of the following problems:**

A. chest pain on rest

B. Chest pain on emotional situations

C.   Severe chest pain associated with evidence of acute heart damage

D.   Heart failure

E.   Heartburn

14.   The following are statements regarding ischemic heart disease:

A.   Reduced coronary blood flow is the main cause

B.   High saturated fat intake is a risk factor

C.   It causes sudden cardiac death

D.   Coagulative necrosis occurs in acute myocardial infarction

E.   It is the leading cause of death worldwide

15.   The following are statements regarding malignant hypertension

A.   It is rapidly progressive end organ damage.

B.   It may complicate any type of hypertension.

C.   There is rapidly developing renal failure.

D.   There is right ventricular failure.

E.   Blood pressure is more than 210/120

16.   The following are statements regarding hypertension:

A.   It is sustained increase in blood pressure

B.   Most of cases are secondary type.

C.   Polycystic kidney disease is etiological factor

D. It may complicate diabetes.

E. Retinopathy is a clinical presentation

17. The following are statements regarding aneurysm

A. False aneurysm is bounded by all the arterial wall components.

B. Fusiform aneurysms involve a long segment of large blood vessels

C. Most abdominal aortic aneurysms are caused by atherosclerosis.

D. In thoracic aortic aneurysms there is dysphagia

E. Circle of Willis is a common location of syphilitic aneurysms.

18. The following are statements regarding aneurysm:

A. Aneurysm is a generalized abnormal dilation of a blood vessel.

B. When a bulging aneurysm is bounded by arterial wall components, it is called a true aneurysm.

C. Arterial dissection arises when blood enters the wall of the artery.

D. Dissections are always aneurysmal.

E. Arterial aneurysms can be caused by systemic diseases

19. The following are statements regarding abdominal aortic aneurysms:

A. Its occurrence is less than thoracic aneurysm.

B. Usually positioned below the renal arteries and above the bibifurcation of the aorta.

C. Inflammatory abdominal aneurysms are not characterized by dense periodic fibrosis.

D. They rarely develop before the age of 50.

E. Clinical course includes embolism from atheroma or mural thrombus.

20. **The following are statements regarding abdominal aortic aneurysm (AAAs)**

A. Abdominal aortic aneurysms are located along the portion of the aorta that passes through the abdomen

B. They are most often seen in women ages 40 to 70 year old.

C. They have been shown to be familial.

D. There is destruction and thinning of the underlying aortic media that has weakened the wall.

E. Inflammatory AAAs are characterized by dense periaortic fibrosis

2.1.b Questions with answers

1.   The following are statements regarding aortic dissection:

T   A.   It may or may not be associated with marked dilatation of the aorta.

T   B.   It can be iatrogenic.

T   C.   It can extend along the aorta toward the heart.

F   D.   In most cases, there is specific underlying preexisting and causal pathology is seen in the aortic wall.

T   E.   Hypertension is clearly the major risk factor overall.

2.   The following are statements regarding aortic dissection:

T   A.   Some dissections are related to the inherited connective tissue disorders.

T   B.   The cause of spontaneous dissections not associated with hypertension is unknown.

F   C.   The classic clinical symptoms are the gradual onset of excruciating pain.

T   D.   The most common cause of death is rupture of the dissection.

F   E.   Myocardial infarction is not common clinical manifestations.

3.   The following are statements regarding rheumatic fever:

F   A.   It follows a Group B beta-hemolytic streptococcal infection.

T   B.   The body produces antibodies that cross react with human tissues.

T   C.   The characteristic lesion of acute rheumatic fever is the Aschoff body

F   D.   The aortic valve is the most affected valve.

T   E.   When pericarditis is present, it rarely affects cardiac function.

4.   The following are statements regarding rheumatic fever:

T   A.   It is acute immunologically mediated.

T   B.   It is multisystem inflammatory disease.

T   C.   It follows an episode of group A srteptococcal pharingitis.

F   D.   It often follows streptococcal infection of skin.

F   E.   It causes chronic deformity of the large joints.

5.   Predisposing factors of cardiac failure include:

T   A.   Coronary blood supply insufficiency.

T   B.   Systemic hypertension.

T   C.   Thyrotoxicosis.

F   D.   Pneumonitis.

T   E.   Diabetes mellitus.

6. Symptoms of heart failure include:

T   A.   Dyspnea

T   B.   Persistent cough

T   C.   Blood tinged sputum

F   D.   Diarrhoea

T   E.   Edema in feet

7. The following are statements regarding Aschoff bodies:

F   A.   They are nodules found in the hearts of individuals with chronic heart disease.

T   B.   Fully developed Aschoff bodies are granulomatous structures consisting of fibrinoid change.

T   C.   They contain lymphocytic infiltration.

T   D.   There are abnormal macrophages surrounding necrotic centers

T   E.   The Aschoff nodules are spheroidal or fusiform distinct tiny structures.

8. Major risk factors of angina pectoris include:

T   A.   Age ($\geq$ 55 years for men, $\geq$ 65 for women)

T   B.   Cigarette smoking

T   C.   Diabetes mellitus

T   D.   Dyslipidemia

T   E.   Hypertension

9. The following are statements regarding infective endocarditis:

F   A.   Gram negative bacilli infect the valves in drug abusers.

F   B.   Prosthetic valves are associated with a lower risk of developing infective endocarditis.

T   C.   Glomerulonephritis is a complication.

T   D.   Vegetations are large and bulky.

T   E.   Vegetations may extend to the chordate tendinae.

10. The following are statements regarding pulmonary vascular diseases:

F   A.   Heart failure cells are seen in pulmonary thromboembolism

T   B.   Pulmonary venous hypertension is caused by congestive heart failure.

T   C.   Adult respiratory distress syndrome can be a complication of sepsis.

F   D.   Cor pulmonale is acute left heart failure due to systemic hypertension.

T   E.   Recurrent thromboemboli in the lungs lead to pulmonary hypertension

11. The following are statements regarding atherosclerosis:

T   A.   It is a chronic disease that remains asymptomatic for decades

T   B.   Atherosclerotic plaques are rich in extracellular matrix and smooth muscle cells.

T   C.   Unstable plaques are rich in macrophages and foam cells

T   D.   Atherosclerosis affects the entire artery tree

T   E.   Diabetes is a risk factor

12.   Risk factors of atherosclerosis include:

T   A.   High serum concentration of low-density lipoprotein

F   B.   High serum concentration of functioning high density lipoprotein

T   C.   Smoking

T   D.   Hypertension

T   E.   Vitamin B_6 deficiency

13.   Ischemic heart disease presents with any of the following problems:

F   A.   chest pain on rest

T   B.   Chest pain on emotional situations

T   C.   Severe chest pain associated with evidence of acute heart damage

T   D.   Heart failure

T   E.   Heartburn

14.   The following are statements regarding ischemic heart disease:

T   A.   Reduced coronary blood flow is the main cause

T   B.   High saturated fat intake is a risk factor

T   C.   It causes sudden cardiac death

F   D.   Coagulative necrosis occurs in acute myocardial infarction

F   E.   It is the leading cause of death worldwide

15.   The following are statements regarding malignant hypertension

T   A.   It is rapidly progressive end organ damage.

T   B.   It may complicate any type of hypertension.

T   C.   There is rapidly developing renal failure.

F   D.   There is right ventricular failure.

T   E.   Blood pressure is more than 210/120

16.   The following are statements regarding hypertension:

T   A.   It is sustained increase in blood pressure

F   B.   Most of cases are secondary type.

T   C.   Polycystic kidney disease is etiological factor

T   D.   It may complicate diabetes.

T   E.   Retinopathy is a clinical presentation

17.   The following are statements regarding aneurysm

F   A.   False aneurysm is bounded by all the arterial wall components.

T   B.   Fusiform aneurysms involve a long segment of large blood vessels

T   C.   Most abdominal aortic aneurysms are caused by atherosclerosis.

T   D.   In thoracic aortic aneurysms there is dysphagia

F   E.   Circle of Willis is a common location of syphilitic aneurysms.

18.   The following are statements regarding aneurysm:

F   A.   Aneurysm is a generalized abnormal dilation of a blood vessel.

T   B.   When a bulging aneurysm is bounded by arterial wall components, it is called a true aneurysm.

T   C.   Arterial dissection arises when blood enters the wall of the artery.

F   D.   Dissections are always aneurysmal.

T   E.   Arterial aneurysms can be caused by systemic diseases

19.   The following are statements regarding abdominal aortic aneurysms:

F   A.   Its occurrence is less than thoracic aneurysm.

T   B.   Usually positioned below the renal arteries and above the bibifurcation of the aorta.

F   C.   Inflammatory abdominal aneurysms are not characterized by dense periodic fibrosis.

T   D.   They rarely develop before the age of 50.

T   E.   Clinical course includes embolism from atheroma or mural thrombus.

20. **The following are statements regarding abdominal aortic aneurysm (AAAs)**

T   A.   Abdominal aortic aneurysms are located along the portion of the aorta that passes through the abdomen

F   B.   They are most often seen in women ages 40 to 70 year old.

T   C.   They have been shown to be familial.

T   D.   There is destruction and thinning of the underlying aortic media that has weakened the wall.

T   E.   Inflammatory AAAs are characterized by dense periaortic fibrosis

2.2 Microbiology of Cardiovascular System

2.2.a Questions without answers

1. **The following are statements regarding infective endocarditis:**

    A.   Higher incidence of the disease is found in patients with congenital heart disease.

    B.   Fever and cardiac murmur are the major presentations.

    C.   One set of blood culture should be taken after initiation of antibiotic therapy.

    D.   Viridans *Streptococcus* is the commonest organism in intravenous drug user.

    E.   Combination of penicillin and aminoglycoside is one of the antibiotic regimens.

2. **Culture-negative infective endocarditis**

    A.   may be due to incorrect clinical diagnosis.

    B.   is only seen in patients with rheumatic heart disease.

    C.   does not present with fever or cardiac murmur.

    D.   can be caused by HACEK group of organisms.

    E.   is usually diagnosed by serological tests.

3.   **Infective endocarditis in injecting drug users**

   A.   usually affects the mitral valve.

   B.   is commonly caused by *Staphylococcus aureus*.

   C.   can be polymicrobial in nature.

   D.   is associated with multiple pulmonary septic emboli.

   E.   is treated with a combination of cloxacillin and gentamicin for 4-6 weeks.

4.   **Basic principles of antibiotic prophylaxis in infective endocarditis include**

   A.   Any bacteriostatic antibiotics can be used.

   B.   The first dose of antibiotic should be given 24 hours before dental procedure.

   C.   Antibiotic prophylaxis should be continued for at least 72 hours.

   D.   Azithromycin is given as an alternative for those allergic to penicillin.

   E.   For patients who have already received penicillin, the use of clindamycin is indicated.

5.   **The following are statements regarding the pathogenesis of sepsis and sepsis-related disorders:**

   A.   Endotoxin is a potent stimulus for the production of cytokines.

B. LPS-binding protein found in the serum neutralizes the effects of endotoxin.

C. Disseminated intravascular coagulation occurs following consumption of platelets.

D. Neutrophils release lysozymes which damage the endothelium.

E. Expression of intracellular adhesion molecules is grossly inhibited.

2.2.b Questions with answers

1. **The following are statements regarding infective endocarditis:**

T   A.   Higher incidence of the disease is found in patients with congenital heart disease.

T   B.   Fever and cardiac murmur are the major presentations.

F   C.   One set of blood culture should be taken after initiation of antibiotic therapy.

F   D.   Viridans *Streptococcus* is the commonest organism in intravenous drug user.

T   E.   Combination of penicillin and aminoglycoside is one of the antibiotic regimens.

2. **Culture-negative infective endocarditis**

T   A.   may be due to incorrect clinical diagnosis.

F   B.   is only seen in patients with rheumatic heart disease.

F   C.   does not present with fever or cardiac murmur.

T   D.   can be caused by HACEK group of organisms.

T   E.   is usually diagnosed by serological tests.

3. **Infective endocarditis in injecting drug users**

F   A.   usually affects the mitral valve.

T   B.   is commonly caused by *Staphylococcus aureus*.

T   C.   can be polymicrobial in nature.

T   D.   is associated with multiple pulmonary septic emboli.

T   E.   is treated with a combination of cloxacillin and gentamicin
         for 4-6 weeks.

4. **Basic principles of antibiotic prophylaxis in infective
    endocarditis include**

F   A.   Any bacteriostatic antibiotics can be used.

F   B.   The first dose of antibiotic should be given 24 hours before
         dental procedure.

F   C.   Antibiotic prophylaxis should be continued for at least 72
         hours.

T   D.   Azithromycin is given as an alternative for those allergic to
         penicillin.

T   E.   For patients who have already received penicillin, the use
         of clindamycin is indicated.

5. **The following are statements regarding the pathogenesis of
    sepsis and sepsis-related disorders:**

T   A.   Endotoxin is a potent stimulus for the production of
         cytokines.

F   B.   LPS-binding protein found in the serum neutralizes the effects of endotoxin.

T   C.   Disseminated intravascular coagulation occurs following consumption of platelets.

T   D.   Neutrophils release lysozymes which damage the endothelium.

F   E.   Expression of intracellular adhesion molecules is grossly inhibited.

3 RESPIRATORY SYSTEM

3.1 Pathology of Respiratory System

3.1.a Questions without answers

1.   **The following are statements regarding lung malignancy:**

   A.   Adenocarcinoma is more common in men compared to women

   B.   Peripheral adenocarcinoma is seen more in non-smokers

   C.   Small cell carcinoma carries a good prognosis

   D.   Cough is the most common presentation

   E.   Squamous cell carcinomas is mostly peripheral in location

2.   **Etiological factors for lung malignancy include:**

   A.   Cigarette smoking

   B.   Radiation

   C.   Benzene exposure

   D.   Asbestos

E.   Intravenous heroin abuse

3.   **The following are statements regarding histological types of lung cancers**

A.   The vast majority of lung cancers are carcinomas

B.   Squamous cell carcinoma usually originates in peripheral lung tissue

C.   Adenocarcinoma of lung typically occurs close to large airways.

D.   In small-cell lung carcinoma, the cells contain dense neurosecretory granules

E.   Most cases of small-cell lung carcinoma arise in the larger airways

4.   **The following are statements regarding pulmonary edema**

A.   It causes pulmonary failure

B.   It is due to either failure of the left ventricle of the heart

C.   Coughing frothy sputum is a symptom

D.   Congested skin is a symptom

E.   Chest X-ray helps in diagnosis

5.   **Causes of pulmonary fibrosis include:**

A.   Asbestosis

B.   Coal miners

    C.   Hypersensitivity pneumonitis

    D.   Cigarette smoking

    E.   Radiation therapy to the chest

6. **Causes of interstitial lung disease include:**

    A.   Silicosis

    B.   Hypersensitivity pneumonitis

    C.   Oral hypoglycemic drugs

    D.   Systemic sclerosis

    E.   Systemic lupus erythematosus

7. **The following are statements regarding bronchopneumonia**

    A.   It is characterized by multiple foci of isolated, acute consolidation, affecting one or more pulmonary lobules.

    B.   It is more likely than lobar pneumonia to be associated with Streptococcus

    C.   It is associated with hospital-acquired pneumonia.

    D.   Presented as multiple foci of consolidation are present in the basal lobes of the lung

    E.   Massive congestion is present

8. **The following are statements regarding lobar pneumonia**

    A.   It is usually caused by aspiration of gastric contents.

    B.   It usually affects infants.

C.   It is usually caused by *Streptococcus pneumoniae*.

D.   It contains neutrophils in alveolar space.

E.   It is rarely associated with the production of sputum.

9.   The following are statements regarding lung abscess

A.   There is necrosis of the pulmonary tissue.

B.   The pus-filled cavity is often caused by aspiration

C.   Alcoholism is the most common condition predisposing factor.

D.   Majority of cases are caused by Aspergillus infection

E.   Night sweats are often presentation

10.   Microscopic findings of pulmonary tuberculosis include

A.   Granuloma

B.   Langerhans giant cells

C.   Lymphocytes

D.   Plasma cells

E.   Fibroblasts with collagen

11.   The following are statements regarding asthma

A.   It is characterized by irreversible bronchospasm.

B.   Extrinsic asthma is classic example of Type I IgE mediated hypersensitivity reaction.

C. Atopic asthma is the most common type of asthma.

D. Acute/intermediate response is bronchoconstriction, edema, mucus secretion, and hypotension.

E. Clinically, it is manifested by episodic dyspnea, cough, and wheezing.

12. **The following are statements regarding emphysema**

A. Acinar and airspace enlargement is usually due to tobacco related wall destruction.

B. Centriacinar emphysema causes significant airflow obstruction.

C. With advanced disease, adjacent alveoli become confluent, creating large airspaces.

D. The lung is pale and voluminous in centriacinar emphysema

E. In centriacinar emphysema the lower two thirds of the lungs is more severely affected than the upper lungs.

13. **The following are statements regarding morphology of emphysema:**

A. In Panacinar emphysema, when well developed, produces pale, voluminous lungs.

B. In Centriacinar emphysema, the lungs are a deeper pink than in panacinar and less voluminous.

C. In extreme cases emphysematous bullae may be grossly visible.

D. Thickening of alveolar walls is histological finding

E. The number of alveolar capillaries is diminished

14.   The following are statements regarding chronic bronchitis:

A.   It is a syndrome of a persistent productive cough for at least 3 consecutive months in at least 2 consecutive years.

B.   Chronic bacterial infection is the major cause

C.   In simple chronic bronchitis, the productive cough raises mucoid sputum, but airflow is not obstructed.

D.   In chronic asthmatic bronchitis, patients demonstrate hyperresponsive airways and intermittent episods of asthma

E.   In chronic obstructive bronchitis, patients develop chronic outflow obstruction.

15.   The following are statements regarding morphology of chronic bronchitis:

A.   The mucosal lining of the larger airways is usually hyperemic and swollen by edema fluid

B.   The smaller bronchi and bronchioles are empty from secretions.

C.   Mucous gland enlargement is the histologic diagnostic hallmark.

D.   The inflammatory cells are mainly neutrophils.

E.   Squamous metaplasia is present.

16.   The following are statements regarding bronchiectasis:

A.   It is a perminant dilition of bronchi and bronchioles.

B.   It is always a primary disease.

C.   Diagnosis depends on an appropriate history along with radiographic demonstration of bronchial dilation.

D.   It can complicate atopic asthma.

E.   Obstruction and chronic persistent infection are critical features in pathogenesis.

17.   **The following are statements regarding morphology of bronchiectasis:**

A.   Usually, affects the upper lobs bilaterally

B.   Usually, the most severe involvement is found in the more distal bronchi and bronchioles

C.   The desquamation of lining epithelium cause extensive areas of ulceration.

D.   Fibrosis of the bronchial and bronchiolar walls.

E.   The necrosis may destroy the bronchial or bronchiolar walls and forms a lung abscess.

18.   **The following are statements regarding pulmonary vascular disease**

A.   Congestive heart failure is the cause of pulmonary arterial hypertension

B.   Autoimmune disease is the cause of pulmonary venous hypertension.

C.   Pulmonary embolism is commonly can be a large bubble of air.

D.   Chronic thromboembolic disease, occurs slowly, and gradually affects a large part of the pulmonary arterial system.

E. A sudden, large pulmonary embolism blocking a large pulmonary artery can cause severe shortness of breath

19. The following are statements regarding pulmonary hypertension

A. It is an increase of blood pressure in the pulmonary artery, pulmonary vein, or pulmonary capillaries.

B. Symptoms develop suddenly.

C. Productive cough is a symptom

D. Pulmonary venous hypertension typically presents with orthopnea

E. The disease might be familial

20. The following are statements regarding carcinoma of lung:

A. Adenocarcinoma is seen frequently in women

B. Squamous cell carcinoma is associated with mucin production in tumor cells.

C. Asbestos exposure is a risk factor.

D. Hypercalcemia occurs as a paraneoplastic syndrome

E. Hoarseness of voice is due to tumor invading the phrenic nerve.

3.1.b Questions with answers

1.   The following are statements regarding lung malignancy:

F   A.   Adenocarcinoma is more common in men compared to women

T   B.   Peripheral adenocarcinoma is seen more in non-smokers

F   C.   Small cell carcinoma carries a good prognosis

T   D.   Cough is the most common presentation

F   E.   Squamous cell carcinomas is mostly peripheral in location

2.   Etiological factors for lung malignancy include:

T   A.   Cigarette smoking

T   B.   Radiation

F   C.   Benzene exposure

T   D.   Asbestos

F   E.   Intravenous heroin abuse

3.   The following are statements regarding histological types of lung cancers

T   A.   The vast majority of lung cancers are carcinomas

F   B.   Squamous cell carcinoma usually originates in peripheral lung tissue

F   C.   Adenocarcinoma of lung typically occurs close to large airways.

T   D.   In small-cell lung carcinoma, the cells contain dense neurosecretory granules

T   E.   Most cases of small-cell lung carcinoma arise in the larger airways

4.   The following are statements regarding pulmonary edema

T   A.   It causes pulmonary failure

T   B.   It is due to either failure of the left ventricle of the heart

T   C.   Coughing frothy sputum is a symptom

F   D.   Congested skin is a symptom

T   E.   Chest X-ray helps in diagnosis

5.   Causes of pulmonary fibrosis include:

T   A.   Asbestosis

T   B.   Coal miners

T   C.   Hypersensitivity pneumonitis

T   D.   Cigarette smoking

T   E.   Radiation therapy to the chest

6.   Causes of interstitial lung disease include:

T   A.   Silicosis

T   B.   Hypersensitivity pneumonitis

F   C.   Oral hypoglycemic drugs

T   D.   Systemic sclerosis

T   E.   Systemic lupus erythematosus

7.   The following are statements regarding bronchopneumonia

T   A.   It is characterized by multiple foci of isolated, acute consolidation, affecting one or more pulmonary lobules.

F   B.   It is more likely than lobar pneumonia to be associated with Streptococcus

T   C.   It is associated with hospital-acquired pneumonia.

T   D.   Presented as multiple foci of consolidation are present in the basal lobes of the lung

T   E.   Massive congestion is present

8.   The following are statements regarding lobar pneumonia

F   A.   It is usually caused by aspiration of gastric contents.

F   B.   It usually affects infants.

T   C.   It is usually caused by *Streptococcus pneumoniae.*

T   D.   It contains neutrophils in alveolar space.

T   E.   It is rarely associated with the production of sputum.

9.   The following are statements regarding lung abscess

T   A.   There is necrosis of the pulmonary tissue.

T   B.   The pus-filled cavity is often caused by aspiration

T   C.   Alcoholism is the most common condition predisposing factor.

F   D.   Majority of cases are caused by Aspergillus infection

T   E.   Night sweats are often presentation

10.   Microscopic findings of pulmonary tuberculosis include

T   A.   Granuloma

T   B.   Langerhans giant cells

T   C.   Lymphocytes

T   D.   Plasma cells

T   E.   Fibroblasts with collagen

11.   The following are statements regarding asthma

F   A.   It is characterized by irreversible bronchospasm.

T   B.   Extrinsic asthma is classic example of Type I IgE mediated hypersensitivity reaction.

T   C.   Atopic asthma is the most common type of asthma.

T   D.   Acute/intermediate response is bronchoconstriction, edema, mucus secretion, and hypotension.

T   E.   Clinically, it is manifested by episodic dyspnea, cough, and wheezing.

12.   The following are statements regarding emphysema

T   A.   Acinar and airspace enlargement is usually due to tobacco related wall destruction.

T   B.   Centriacinar emphysema causes significant airflow obstruction.

T   C.   With advanced disease, adjacent alveoli become confluent, creating large airspaces.

F   D.   The lung is pale and voluminous in centriacinar emphysema

F   E.   In centriacinar emphysema the lower two thirds of the lungs is more severely affected than the upper lungs.

13.   The following are statements regarding morphology of emphysema:

T   A.   In Panacinar emphysema, when well developed, produces pale, voluminous lungs.

T   B.   In Centriacinar emphysema, the lungs are a deeper pink than in panacinar and less voluminous.

T   C.   In extreme cases emphysematous bullae may be grossly visible.

F   D.   Thickening of alveolar walls is histological finding

T   E.   The number of alveolar capillaries is diminished

14.   The following are statements regarding chronic bronchitis:

T   A.   It is a syndrome of a persistent productive cough for at least 3 consecutive months in at least 2 consecutive years.

F   B.   Chronic bacterial infection is the major cause

T   C.   In simple chronic bronchitis, the productive cough raises mucoid sputum, but airflow is not obstructed.

T   D.   In chronic asthmatic bronchitis, patients demonstrate hyperresponsive airways and intermittent episods of asthma

T   E.   In chronic obstructive bronchitis, patients develop chronic outflow obstruction.

15. The following are statements regarding morphology of chronic bronchitis:

T   A.   The mucosal lining of the larger airways is usually hyperemic and swollen by edema fluid

F   B.   The smaller bronchi and bronchioles are empty from secretions.

T   C.   Mucous gland enlargement is the histologic diagnostic hallmark.

F   D.   The inflammatory cells are mainly neutrophils.

T   E.   Squamous metaplasia is present.

16. The following are statements regarding bronchiectasis:

T   A.   It is a perminant dilition of bronchi and bronchioles.

F   B.   It is always a primary disease.

T   C.   Diagnosis depends on an appropriate history along with radiographic demonstration of bronchial dilation.

T   D.   It can complicate atopic asthma.

T   E.   Obstruction and chronic persistent infection are critical features in pathogenesis.

17. The following are statements regarding morphology of bronchiectasis:

F   A.   Usually, affects the upper lobs bilaterally

T   B.   Usually, the most severe involvement is found in the more distal bronchi and bronchioles

T   C.   The desquamation of lining epithelium cause extensive areas of ulceration.

T   D.   Fibrosis of the bronchial and bronchiolar walls.

T   E.   The necrosis may destroy the bronchial or bronchiolar walls and forms a lung abscess.

18. The following are statements regarding pulmonary vascular disease

F   A.   Congestive heart failure is the cause of pulmonary arterial hypertension

F   B.   Autoimmune disease is the cause of pulmonary venous hypertension.

F   C.   Pulmonary embolism is commonly can be a large bubble of air.

T   D.   Chronic thromboembolic disease, occurs slowly, and gradually affects a large part of the pulmonary arterial system.

T   E.   A sudden, large pulmonary embolism blocking a large pulmonary artery can cause severe shortness of breath

19. The following are statements regarding pulmonary hypertension

T   A.   It is an increase of blood pressure in the pulmonary artery, pulmonary vein, or pulmonary capillaries.

F   B.   Symptoms develop suddenly.

F   C.   Productive cough is a symptom

T   D.   Pulmonary venous hypertension typically presents with orthopnea

T   E.   The disease might be familial

20.   The following are statements regarding carcinoma of lung:

T   A.   Adenocarcinoma is seen frequently in women

F   B.   Squamous cell carcinoma is associated with mucin production in tumor cells.

T   C.   Asbestos exposure is a risk factor.

T   D.   Hypercalcemia occurs as a paraneoplastic syndrome

F   E.   Hoarseness of voice is due to tumor invading the phrenic nerve.

3.2 Microbiology of Respiratory System

3.2.a Questions without answers

1. **The following are statements regarding Legionnaires' disease:**

    A.   It commonly affects the middle-aged, male, chronic smokers.

    B.   Inhalation of contaminated aerosols from the cooling towers is the mode of transmission.

    C.   The causative organism is a Gram-positive bacillus which grows on Bordet- Gengou agar.

    D.   Diagnosis is made by four-fold rise in antibody titre by microagglutination test.

    E.   A combination of cefotaxime and metronidazole is used in the treatment.

2. **The following are statements regarding bacterial pneumonia:**

    A.   It is often preceded by viral upper respiratory tract infections.

    B.   *Streptococcus pneumoniae* is a common cause of aspiration pneumonia.

C.   High grade fever with productive cough is the common clinical manifestation.

D.   Majority of the causative agents of atypical pneumonia are easily cultured.

E.   Penicillin is the antibiotic of choice for pneumonia caused by *Mycoplasma pneumoniae.*

3.   **Pertussis**

A.   is commonly caused by *Bordetella parapertussis.*

B.   is due to the toxin released by the causative organism.

C.   may cause cerebral anoxia as a complication.

D.   is also common in birds.

E.   is prevented by a subunit vaccine.

4.   **Diphtheria**

A.   is caused by all strains of *Corynebacterium diphtheriae.*

B.   is due to the exotoxin released by the causative organism.

C.   is characterized by the presence of pseudomembrane over the pharynx.

D.   results in myocarditis and polyneuritis as complications.

E.   can be prevented by a killed vaccine.

5. **Acute bronchiolitis**

   A.   mainly affects children above the age of 5 years.

   B.   is commonly caused by Epstein-Barr virus.

   C.   presents with wheezing and intercosal recession.

   D.   can be diagnosed clinically.

   E.   is treated with oxygen and nebulized tribavirin.

6. **The following are statements regarding common cold:**

   A.   Rhinoviruses and coronaviruses are among the common causative agents.

   B.   Low grade fever, nasal stuffiness and runny nose are common clinical manifestations.

   C.   Transmission is via direct contact with infected respiratory secretions.

   D.   Diagnosis is only confirmed by culture of sputum.

   E.   Anti-viral therapy is required in majority of cases.

7. **The frequency of influenza epidemics is associated with**

   A.   the frequent mutations in viral genes for the envelope glycoproteins.

   B.   numerous animal and human carriers.

   C.   wide variety of virus families that can cause influenza.

   D.   ability of the influenza virus to be transmitted via contaminated public water supplies.

E.   lack of available immunization.

8   **The following are pairs regarding the respiratory viruses and their associated infections:**

A.   Influenza A   :   Primary viral pneumonia.

B.   Parainfluenza virus   :   SARS.

C.   Measles   :   Giant cell pneumonia in immunocompromised host.

D.   Adenovirus   :   Pharyngoconjunctival fever.

E.   Cytomegalovirus   :   Heterophile-positive infectious mononucleosis.

9.   **The following are statements regarding tuberculosis:**

A.   The causative organism grows rapidly on Lowenstein-Jensen medium.

B.   Primary complex consists of the Ghon focus and marked enlargement of the hilar lymph nodes.

C.   The pulmonary lesion is almost always at the apex in primary tuberculosis.

D.   Cavitation is due to destruction of lung tissue by toxins released by *Mycobacterium tuberculosis*.

E.   Direct observed treatment short course (DOTS) is its highly effective treatment in developing countries.

10. **The following are statements regarding diagnosis and treatment of tuberculosis :**

   A. Positive Mantoux test indicates an active disease.

   B. Sputum is cultured on Lowenstein-Jensen medium and incubated for 4-6 weeks.

   C. Combined antibiotic therapy is required to prevent rapid emergence of resistance in the causative agent.

   D. Drug-resistant tuberculosis is treated with high doses of rifampicin or isoniazid.

   E. Advantages of DOTS (Direct Observed Treatment, short course) include

   high cure rate and no necessity for hospitalization.

3.2.b Questions with answers

1. The following are statements regarding Legionnaires' disease:

T A. It commonly affects the middle-aged, male, chronic smokers.

T B. Inhalation of contaminated aerosols from the cooling towers is the mode of transmission.

F C. The causative organism is a Gram-positive bacillus which grows on Bordet- Gengou agar.

T D. Diagnosis is made by four-fold rise in antibody titre by microagglutination test.

F E. A combination of cefotaxime and metronidazole is used in the treatment.

2. The following are statements regarding bacterial pneumonia:

T A. It is often preceded by viral upper respiratory tract infections.

F B. *Streptococcus pneumoniae* is a common cause of aspiration pneumonia.

T C. High grade fever with productive cough is the common clinical manifestation.

F   D.   Majority of the causative agents of atypical pneumonia are easily cultured.

F   E.   Penicillin is the antibiotic of choice for pneumonia caused by *Mycoplasma pneumoniae.*

3. Pertussis

F   A.   is commonly caused by *Bordetella parapertussis.*

T   B.   is due to the toxin released by the causative organism.

T   C.   may cause cerebral anoxia as a complication.

F   D.   is also common in birds.

T   E.   is prevented by a subunit vaccine.

4. Diphtheria

F   A.   is caused by all strains of *Corynebacterium diphtheriae.*

T   B.   is due to the exotoxin released by the causative organism.

T   C.   is characterized by the presence of pseudomembrane over the pharynx.

T   D.   results in myocarditis and polyneuritis as complications.

F   E.   can be prevented by a killed vaccine.

5. Acute bronchiolitis

F   A.   mainly affects children above the age of 5 years.

F   B.   is commonly caused by Epstein-Barr virus.

T   C.   presents with wheezing and intercosal recession.

T   D.   can be diagnosed clinically.

T   E.   is treated with oxygen and nebulized tribavirin.

6.   The following are statements regarding common cold:

T   A.   Rhinoviruses and coronaviruses are among the common causative agents.

T   B.   Low grade fever, nasal stuffiness and runny nose are common clinical manifestations.

T   C.   Transmission is via direct contact with infected respiratory secretions.

F   D.   Diagnosis is only confirmed by culture of sputum.

F   E.   Anti-viral therapy is required in majority of cases.

7.   The frequency of influenza epidemics is associated with

T   A.   the frequent mutations in viral genes for the envelope glycoproteins.

F   B.   numerous animal and human carriers.

F   C.   wide variety of virus families that can cause influenza.

F   D.   ability of the influenza virus to be transmitted via contaminated public water supplies.

F   E.   lack of available immunization.

8   **The following are pairs regarding the respiratory viruses and their associated infections:**

T   A.   Influenza A   :   Primary viral pneumonia.

F   B.   Parainfluenza virus   :   SARS.

T   C.   Measles   :   Giant cell pneumonia in immunocompromised host.

T   D.   Adenovirus   :   Pharyngoconjunctival fever.

F   E.   Cytomegalovirus   :   Heterophile-positive infectious mononucleosis.

9.   **The following are statements regarding tuberculosis:**

T   A.   The causative organism grows rapidly on Lowenstein-Jensen medium.

T   B.   Primary complex consists of the Ghon focus and marked enlargement of the hilar lymph nodes.

F   C.   The pulmonary lesion is almost always at the apex in primary tuberculosis.

F   D.   Cavitation is due to destruction of lung tissue by toxins released by *Mycobacterium tuberculosis*.

T   E.   Direct observed treatment short course (DOTS) is its highly effective treatment in developing countries.

10.   **The following are statements regarding diagnosis and treatment of tuberculosis :**

F   A.   Positive Mantoux test indicates an active disease.

T   B.   Sputum is cultured on Lowenstein-Jensen medium and incubated for 4-6 weeks.

T   C.   Combined antibiotic therapy is required to prevent rapid emergence of resistance in the causative agent.

F   D.   Drug-resistant tuberculosis is treated with high doses of rifampicin or isoniazid.

T   E.   Advantages of DOTS (Direct Observed Treatment, short course) include

high cure rate and no necessity for hospitalization.

4 MUSCULOSKELETAL SYSTEM

4.1 Pathology of Musculoskeletal System

4.1.a Questions without answers

1.   The following are statements regarding osteoporosis

A.   Cushing's syndrome is associated with osteoporosis

B.   The level of estrogen increases in these patients

C.   Low serum calcium is a finding.

D.   It is common in post menopausal women

E.   Kyphosis is one of the complications

2.   The following are statements regarding Rickets, Osteomalacia and Hyperparathyroidism:

A.   In patients with rickets rickety rosary is seen in the long bones

B.   Vitamin D deficiency causes rickets in children

C.   Vitamin A deficiency in adults is the cause of the formation of thick osteoid

D.   Pathological fractures occur commonly in hyporparathyroidism

E.   Histologically, the brown tumor of hyperparathyroidism shows osteoclasts and haemorrhage

3.   Risk factors of osteoporosis include:

A.   Oestrogen deficiency following menopause

B.   Tobacco smoking

C.   Vitamin D deficiency

D.   Being overweight

E.   Soft drinks

4.   Regarding osteomyelitis (OM)

A.   Chronic osteomyelitis may be due to the presence of intracellular bacteria (inside bone cells)

B.   Areas of necrotic bone are the basis for distinguishing between acute OM and chronic.

C.   In adults OM, large subperiosteal abscesses can form.

D.   Staphylococcus aureus is the organism most commonly isolated from all forms of osteomyelitis

E.   Radiology is diagnostic.

5.   The following are statements regarding myasthenia gravis

A.   It is an autoimmune disease

B.   The hallmark of myasthenia gravis is fatigability

C.   The onset of the disorder can be sudden

D.   In most cases, the first noticeable symptom is weakness of the eye muscles

E.   Serological tests for antibodies are diagnostic for all cases

6.   **The following are statements regarding spinal muscular atrophy**

A.   It is an autosomal dominant disease

B.   It is the most common genetic cause of infant death.

C.   Areflexia, particularly in extremities is a presentation

D.   Baby born with weight lower than normal

E.   Prenatal screening is controversial

7.   **The following are statements regarding skin tumor**

A.   Melanoma is the most serious type.

B.   Basal and squamous cell cancer are the two most common types of skin cancer.

C.   Ultraviolet light is the most important factor especially in those with fair skin.

D.   Dysplastic nevi and large congenital nevus are premalignant

E.   Basal cell carcinomas are present on sun-exposed areas of the skin, especially the face.

8. **The following are statements regarding skin tumor**

   A. Squamous cell cancer originates from the lowest layer of the epidermis

   B. Melanoma is the least common, but most aggressive.

   C. Basal cell carcinoma morphology; the pearly translucency to fleshy color, tiny blood vessels on the surface, and sometime ulceration which can be characteristics.

   D. Basal cell carcinomas are present on sun-exposed areas of the skin, especially the face.

   E. Change in the size, shape, color or elevation of a mole are warning signs of malignant melanoma

9. **The following are statements regarding soft tissue sarcoma**

   A. They are relatively common cancers

   B. They usually cause symptoms in their early stages

   C. A painless lump or swelling is the first noticeable symptom

   D. Biopsy is diagnostic.

   E. Lungs are the most common site to which soft tissue sarcoma spreads

10. **The following are statements regarding lipoma**

   A. It is a malignant tumor composed of adipose tissue

   B. Lipomas are commonly found in children

   C. Adenolipomas are lipomas associated with eccrine sweat glands

D. Lipomas are usually relatively small with diameters of about 1–3 cm.

E. Familial multiple lipomatosis is a leading cause

11. **The following are statements regarding giant cell tumour of bone:**

A. It is usually arise from the epiphysis of long bone

B. It shows soap bubble appearance on X-Rays

C. It is generally malignant in behavior

D. It is common in children.

E. Its prognosis is dependent upon the number of osteoclastic giant cells.

12. **The following are statements regarding bone neoplasms:**

A. Osteoma is cartilage forming tumour

B. Osteosarcoma affects the metaphyseal area

C. Chondrosarcoma typically affects children

D. Ewing sarcoma consists of small cells on histology

E. Giant cell tumour is seen characteristically around the knee

13. **The following are statements regarding bone tumors:**

A. Primary bone tumour are more common than secondary malignant tumour

B.   Breast carcinoma commonly metastasizes to the bone

C.   Osteogenic sarcoma shows sunburst appearance on X- Ray

D.   Ewing sarcoma commonly occurs in the elderly

E.   Chondrosarcoma commonly occurs in children

14.   Osteosarcoma

A.   is common in the elderly age group

B.   is associated with trauma

C.   arises from the metaphyseal region of long bones

D.   is histologically characterised by the presence of osteoid and pleomorphism of tumour cells

E.   is associated with Paget's disease of bone

15.   Skeletal metastasis is characteristically seen in

A.   glioblastoma multiforme

B.   thyroid carcinoma

C.   breast carcinoma

D.   lung carcinoma

E.   nasopharyngeal carcinoma

16.   The following are statements regarding osteosarcoma

A.   It is common in adolescents

B.   If occur in elderly, it is associated with worse prognosis

C.   Chondrosarcoma typically affects children

D.   Ewing sarcoma consists of small cells on histology

E.   Giant cell tumour is seen characteristically around the knee

17.   The following are statements regarding rheumatoid arthritis:

A.   It is an autoimmune disease that affects many tissues and organs.

B.   It is monoarthritis disease.

C.   There is a genetic link with HLA-DR4 and the disease

D.   X-rays of the hands and feet are generally performed to the patients.

E.   A negative rheumatoid factor is enough to exclude the disease

18.   The following are statements regarding arthritic bone diseases

A.   Pannus formation is a characteristic feature of rheumatoid arthritis

B.   Rice bodies are seen in osteoarthritis

C.   Fibrinoid necrosis is seen in rheumatoid nodules

D.   The shoulder joint is the commonest site of attack of gouty arthritis.

E.   Tophaceous deposits of urate are common in the brain

19.   The following are statements regarding gout

A.   It is a cause of kidney stones

B.   Heart diseases are a risk factor.

C.   It is associated with low uric acid level in blood

D.   Sea food is a risk factor

E.   The formation of tophi in the central nervous system is a complication.

20.   **The following are statements regarding osteoporosis**

A.   It is characterized by low bone mass

B.   Being male is a risk factor

C.   The hallmark of osteoporosis is the loss of bone

D.   There is thinning of the trabeculae and widening of haversian canals.

E.   Osteoclastic activity is present but is not increased in microscopic sections.

4.1.b Questions with answers

1. The following are statements regarding osteoporosis

T   A.   Cushing's syndrome is associated with osteoporosis

F   B.   The level of estrogen increases in these patients

F   C.   Low serum calcium is a finding.

T   D.   It is common in post menopausal women

T   E.   Kyphosis is one of the complications

2. The following are statements regarding Rickets, Osteomalacia and Hyperparathyroidism:

F   A.   In patients with rickets rickety rosary is seen in the long bones

T   B.   Vitamin D deficiency causes rickets in children

F   C.   Vitamin A deficiency in adults is the cause of the formation of thick osteoid

F   D.   Pathological fractures occur commonly in hyporparathyroidism

T   E.   Histologically, the brown tumor of hyperparathyroidism shows osteoclasts and haemorrhage

3. Risk factors of osteoporosis include:

T   A.   Oestrogen deficiency following menopause

T   B.   Tobacco smoking

T   C.   Vitamin D deficiency

F   D.   Being overweight

T   E.   Soft drinks

4. Regarding osteomyelitis (OM)

T   A.   Chronic osteomyelitis may be due to the presence of intracellular bacteria (inside bone cells)

T   B.   Areas of necrotic bone are the basis for distinguishing between acute OM and chronic.

F   C.   In adults OM, large subperiosteal abscesses can form.

T   D.   Staphylococcus aureus is the organism most commonly isolated from all forms of osteomyelitis

T   E.   Radiology is diagnostic.

5. The following are statements regarding myasthenia gravis

T   A.   It is an autoimmune disease

T   B.   The hallmark of myasthenia gravis is fatigability

T   C.   The onset of the disorder can be sudden

T   D.   In most cases, the first noticeable symptom is weakness of the eye muscles

F   E.   Serological tests for antibodies are diagnostic for all cases

6. **The following are statements regarding spinal muscular atrophy**

F   A.   It is an autosomal dominant disease

T   B.   It is the most common genetic cause of infant death.

T   C.   Areflexia, particularly in extremities is a presentation

T   D.   Baby born with weight lower than normal

T   E.   Prenatal screening is controversial

7. **The following are statements regarding skin tumor**

T   A.   Melanoma is the most serious type.

T   B.   Basal and squamous cell cancer are the two most common types of skin cancer.

T   C.   Ultraviolet light is the most important factor especially in those with fair skin.

T   D.   Dysplastic nevi and large congenital nevus are premalignant

T   E.   Basal cell carcinomas are present on sun-exposed areas of the skin, especially the face.

8. **The following are statements regarding skin tumor**

F   A.   Squamous cell cancer originates from the lowest layer of the epidermis

T   B.   Melanoma is the least common, but most aggressive.

T   C.   Basal cell carcinoma morphology; the pearly translucency to fleshy color, tiny blood vessels on the surface, and sometime ulceration which can be characteristics.

T   D.   Basal cell carcinomas are present on sun-exposed areas of the skin, especially the face.

T   E.   Change in the size, shape, color or elevation of a mole are warning signs of malignant melanoma

9.   The following are statements regarding soft tissue sarcoma

F   A.   They are relatively common cancers

F   B.   They usually cause symptoms in their early stages

T   C.   A painless lump or swelling is the first noticeable symptom

T   D.   Biopsy is diagnostic.

T   E.   Lungs are the most common site to which soft tissue sarcoma spreads

10.   The following are statements regarding lipoma

T   A.   It is a malignant tumor composed of adipose tissue

F   B.   Lipomas are commonly found in children

T   C.   Adenolipomas are lipomas associated with eccrine sweat glands

T   D.   Lipomas are usually relatively small with diameters of about 1– 3 cm.

T   E.   Familial multiple lipomatosis is a leading cause

11.   The following are statements regarding giant cell tumour of bone:

T   A.   It is usually arise from the epiphysis of long bone

T   B.   It shows soap bubble appearance on X-Rays

F   C.   It is generally malignant in behavior

F   D.   It is common in children.

F   E.   Its prognosis is dependent upon the number of osteoclastic giant cells.

12.   The following are statements regarding bone neoplasms:

F   A.   Osteoma is cartilage forming tumour

T   B.   Osteosarcoma affects the metaphyseal area

F   C.   Chondrosarcoma typically affects children

T   D.   Ewing sarcoma consists of small cells on histology

T   E.   Giant cell tumour is seen characteristically around the knee

13.   The following are statements regarding bone tumors:

F   A.   Primary bone tumour are more common than secondary malignant tumour

T   B.   Breast carcinoma commonly metastasizes to the bone

T   C.   Osteogenic sarcoma shows sunburst appearance on X- Ray

F   D.   Ewing sarcoma commonly occurs in the elderly

F   E.   Chondrosarcoma commonly occurs in children

14.   Osteosarcoma

F   A.   is common in the elderly age group

F   B.   is associated with trauma

T   C.   arises from the metaphyseal region of long bones

T   D.   is histologically characterised by the presence of osteoid and pleomorphism of tumour cells

T   E.   is associated with Paget's disease of bone

15. Skeletal metastasis is characteristically seen in

F   A.   glioblastoma multiforme

T   B.   thyroid carcinoma

T   C.   breast carcinoma

T   D.   lung carcinoma

F   E.   nasopharyngeal carcinoma

16. The following are statements regarding osteosarcoma

T   A.   It is common in adolescents

T   B.   If occur in elderly, it is associated with worse prognosis

F   C.   Chondrosarcoma typically affects children

T   D.   Ewing sarcoma consists of small cells on histology

T   E.   Giant cell tumour is seen characteristically around the knee

17. The following are statements regarding rheumatoid arthritis:

T   A.   It is an autoimmune disease that affects many tissues and organs.

F   B.   It is monoarthritis disease.

T   C.   There is a genetic link with HLA-DR4 and the disease

T   D.   X-rays of the hands and feet are generally performed to the patients.

F   E.   A negative rheumatoid factor is enough to exclude the disease

18. The following are statements regarding arthritic bone diseases

T   A.   Pannus formation is a characteristic feature of rheumatoid arthritis

F   B.   Rice bodies are seen in osteoarthritis

T   C.   Fibrinoid necrosis is seen in rheumatoid nodules

F   D.   The shoulder joint is the commonest site of attack of gouty arthritis.

F   E.   Tophaceous deposits of urate are common in the brain

19. The following are statements regarding gout

T   A.   It is a cause of kidney stones

F   B.   Heart diseases are a risk factor.

F   C.   It is associated with low uric acid level in blood

T   D.   Sea food is a risk factor

F   E.   The formation of tophi in the central nervous system is a complication.

20.   The following are statements regarding osteoporosis

T   A.   It is characterized by low bone mass

F   B.   Being male is a risk factor

T   C.   The hallmark of osteoporosis is the loss of bone

T   D.   There is thinning of the trabeculae and widening of haversian canals.

T   E.   Osteoclastic activity is present but is not increased in microscopic sections.

4.2 Microbiology of Musculoskeletal System

4.2.a Questions without answers

1.   Measles

A.   is caused by an orthomyxovirus.

B.   is characterized by the presence of Koplik's spots on the buccal mucosa.

C.   presents with pneumonia due to a secondary bacterial infection.

D.   confers a short-lived immunity.

E.   antibody can be detected in the cerebrospinal fluid of patients with subacute sclerosing panencephalitis (SSPE).

2.   Rubella

A.   is caused by non-arthropod-borne togavirus.

B.   is transmitted via fecal-oral route.

C.   presents with painful sub-occipital lymph nodes.

D.   which occurs in the 3rd trimester of pregnancy causes congenital infection.

E.   is diagnosed by detecting rubella-specific IgM.

3. **Necrotizing fasciitis**

 A. is a rapidly spreading infection involving subcutaneous tissues.

 B. can be caused by multiple organisms often of the gut origin.

 C. is common in patients with diabetes mellitus.

 D. is associated with untreated toxic shock syndrome.

 E. requires surgical debridement and combined antibiotic therapy.

4. **Scalded skin syndrome**

 A. is a toxin-mediated disease.

 B. is commonly caused by *Streptococcus pyogenes*.

 C. results in toxic shock syndrome if left untreated.

 D. presents with generalized desquamation of the skin.

 E. is treated with cloxacillin.

5. **Gas gangrene**

 A. is caused by *Clostridium perfringens*.

 B. presents with necrosis and gas in the affected tissue.

 C. can be spontaneous as a result of blood-borne spread from colorectal cancer.

D. is diagnosed by the presence of Gram-negative bacilli in direct smear of exudates.

E. requires extensive surgical debridement and antibiotic therapy.

6. **The following are statements regarding acute osteomyelitis:**

A. It can be due to hematogenous spread.

B. In diabetes mellitus, small bones of the feet are commonly affected.

C. Demineralization of bone is seen in the early stages.

D. *Staphylococcus aureus* is the most common causative organism.

E. Presence of sequestrum and involucrum is the characteristic feature.

7. **Reactive arthritis**

A. is commonly caused by *Haemophilus influenzae.*

B. is commonly associated with HLA-B27.

C. is associated with sexually transmitted diseases

D. is usually blood culture-positive.

E. is treated with long-term antibiotics.

8. **Tinea capitis**

A.   is an infection of the scalp and hair by dermatophytes.

B.   can be acquired from household pets.

C.   shows symptoms ranging from mild scaly lesion to alopecia.

D.   is diagnosed by detecting hyphae with budding yeasts in skin scrapings.

E.   is treated with cotrimoxazole.

9.   **Pityriasis versicolor**

A.   is a superficial infection of the stratum corneum.

B.   is commonly caused by *Microsporum* sp.

C.   is spread via contaminated bedding/clothing.

D.   presents with multiple subcutaneous nodules along the lymphatics.

E.   is treated with griseofulvin.

10.   **Sporotrichosis**

A.   is a chronic infection caused by a dimorphic fungus.

B.   is acquired via traumatic inoculation of the skin.

C.   presents with either hyperpigmented or hypopigmented macules on the skin.

D.   is characterized by the presence of steroid bodies in tissues.

E.   is treated with oral itraconazole.

4.2.b Questions with answers

1. Measles

F A. is caused by an orthomyxovirus.

T B. is characterized by the presence of Koplik's spots on the buccal mucosa.

T C. presents with pneumonia due to a secondary bacterial infection.

F D. confers a short-lived immunity.

T E. antibody can be detected in the cerebrospinal fluid of patients with subacute sclerosing panencephalitis (SSPE).

2. Rubella

T A. is caused by non-arthropod-borne togavirus.

F B. is transmitted via fecal-oral route.

T C. presents with painful sub-occipital lymph nodes.

F D. which occurs in the 3rd trimester of pregnancy causes congenital infection.

T E. is diagnosed by detecting rubella-specific IgM.

3.   Necrotizing fasciitis

T   A.   is a rapidly spreading infection involving subcutaneous tissues.

T   B.   can be caused by multiple organisms often of the gut origin.

T   C.   is common in patients with diabetes mellitus.

F   D.   is associated with untreated toxic shock syndrome.

T   E.   requires surgical debridement and combined antibiotic therapy.

4.   Scalded skin syndrome

T   A.   is a toxin-mediated disease.

F   B.   is commonly caused by *Streptococcus pyogenes*.

F   C.   results in toxic shock syndrome if left untreated.

T   D.   presents with generalized desquamation of the skin.

T   E.   is treated with cloxacillin.

5.   Gas gangrene

T   A.   is caused by *Clostridium perfringens*.

T   B.   presents with necrosis and gas in the affected tissue.

T   C.   can be spontaneous as a result of blood-borne spread from colorectal cancer.

F   D.   is diagnosed by the presence of Gram-negative bacilli in direct smear of exudates.

T   E.   requires extensive surgical debridement and antibiotic therapy.

6.   The following are statements regarding acute osteomyelitis:

T   A.   It can be due to hematogenous spread.

T   B.   In diabetes mellitus, small bones of the feet are commonly affected.

F   C.   Demineralization of bone is seen in the early stages.

T   D.   *Staphylococcus aureus* is the most common causative organism.

F   E.   Presence of sequestrum and involucrum is the characteristic feature.

7.   Reactive arthritis

F   A.   is commonly caused by *Haemophilus influenzae*.

T   B.   is commonly associated with HLA-B27.

T   C.   is associated with sexually transmitted diseases

F   D.   is usually blood culture-positive.

F   E.   is treated with long-term antibiotics.

8.   Tinea capitis

T   A.   is an infection of the scalp and hair by dermatophytes.

T   B.   can be acquired from household pets.

T   C.   shows symptoms ranging from mild scaly lesion to alopecia.

F   D.   is diagnosed by detecting hyphae with budding yeasts in skin scrapings.

F   E.   is treated with cotrimoxazole.

9.   Pityriasis versicolor

T   A.   is a superficial infection of the stratum corneum.

F   B.   is commonly caused by *Microsporum* sp.

T   C.   is spread via contaminated bedding/clothing.

F   D.   presents with multiple subcutaneous nodules along the lymphatics.

F   E.   is treated with griseofulvin.

10.   Sporotrichosis

T   A.   is a chronic infection caused by a dimorphic fungus.

T   B.   is acquired via traumatic inoculation of the skin.

F   C.   presents with either hyperpigmented or hypopigmented macules on the skin.

F   D.   is characterized by the presence of steroid bodies in tissues.

T   E.   is treated with oral itraconazole.

5 HEMATOPOIETIC AND LYMPHOID SYSTEM

5.1 Pathology of Hematopoietic and Lymphoid System

5.1.a Questions without answers

1. **The following are statements regarding megaloblastic anaemia**

   A. It is due to inhibition of DNA synthesis in red blood cell production

   B. Blood film shows microcytic red blood cells

   C. Alcohol abuse is one of the causes

   D. Present of nuclear hypersegmentation of neutrophils.

   E. Thrombocytosis is a finding.

2. **The following are statements regarding haemolytic anaemia**

   A. In Microangiopathic Haemolytic Anemia (MAHA) the platelet count is decreased.

   B. Direct Coombs' test is positive in all of non immune cases.

C.   Conjugated bilirubin in the blood is elevated

D.   Sickle cell anaemia is associated with abnormality of RBC membrane.

E.   Blood smear shows elevated numbers of reticulocytes

3.   **The following are statements regarding laboratory changes in anaemia:**

A.   Platelet count is increased in megaloblastic anaemia

B.   Total iron-binding capacity (TIBC) is low in iron deficiency anaemia

C.   There is low thyroid hormone level in some patients

D.   Serum lactate dehydrogenase (LDH) is elevated in haemolytic anaemia

E.   Blood smear show macrocytic changes in anaemia due to chronic blood loss

4.   **The following are statements regarding thalassemia**

A.   It is an inherited autosomal recessive blood disorder

B.   Patient with thalassemia makes more hemoglobin but fewer circulating red blood cells than normal.

C.   Beta thalassemias are due to mutations in the HBB gene on chromosome 11.

D.   Iron supplements are useful in treatment

E.   Pneumonia is a complication

5. **The following are statements regarding Beta-thalassemias**

   A. Patient is usually presented at adolescence age with severe anemia

   B. In thalassemia mainor, only one of β globin alleles bears a mutation

   C. Severe bone deformities is a presentation in thalassemia major

   D. Cure is possible by bone marrow transplantation

   E. Affected patient requires regular lifelong blood transfusions.

6. **The following are statements regarding clotting disorders**

   A. There is thrombocytopenia in laboratory evaluation.

   B. There is prolongation of PT and PTT.

   C. Fibrin split products are increased in the plasma

   D. DIC can be life threatening.

   E. The underlying disorder must not be treated simultaneously.

7. **Coagulation disorders include:**

   A. Hemophilia (A, B).

   B. Von-Willebrand's disease.

   C. Vitamin-K deficiency.

   D. Henoch-Schonlein purpura.

   E. Idiopathic thrombocytopenic purpura (ITP).

8. **Causes of pancytopenia include:**

    A. Multiple myeloma.

    B. Megaloblastic anemia.

    C. Aplastic anemia.

    D. Bone marrow infiltration.

    E. Sickle cell anemia.

9. **Regarding Hemophilia**

    A. Hemophilia A, accounts for about 80% of all cases, is a deficiency in clotting factor IX.

    B. The bleeding patterns and consequences of two types of hemophilia are different.

    C. Petechiae are characteristically absent.

    D. Cephalhematoma is one of characterstic features in infant females

    E. There is prolonged bleeding time.

10. **Effects and complications of bone marrow failure include:**

    A. Normochromic normocytic anemia.

    B. Thrombocytopenia.

    C. Increased susceptibility to infection.

    D. Neutrophilia.

    E. Presence of blast cells in the peripheral blood.

11. The following are statements regarding bone marrow failure

A. Radiations is a cause

B. Patient is susceptible easily to get infection

C. Patient is anemic

D. Bone marrow is hyperplastic

E. Bone marrow aspiration is diagnostic

12. The following are statements regarding aplastic anemia

A. Etiology is idiopathic, in more than half of cases.

B. It increasingly appears that autoreactive B cells play an important role in pathogenesis.

C. Bone marrow typically is markedly hypocellular

D. In BM biopsy specimens; small foci of lymphcytes and plasma cells may be seen.

E. Thrombocytopenia often presents as the appearance of petechiae and ecchymosis.

13. The following are statements regarding chronic myeloid leukemia:

A. Philadelphia chromosome is absent in most of the cases.

B. Neutrophil alkaline phosphatase score is increased.

C. Normochromic normocytic anemia is usual.

D. There is leucocytosis.

E. Basophilia is common.

14. Characteristic features of acute leukaemias include :

A. Children under 15 years most commonly affected in acute lymphoblastic leukemia(ALL)

B. Gum hypertrophy is characteristic in acute lymphoblastic leukemia(ALL)

C. Predominance of lymphoblasts in blood and bone marrow in acute myeloblastic leukemia(AML)

D. Acid phosphatase diffuse positivity in leukaemic blasts in acute lymphoblastic leukemia(ALL)

E. Remission rate is high in acute lymphoblastic leukemia(ALL)

15. The following are statements regarding chronic myeloid leukemia

A. The blast cells in peripheral blood smear are increased more than 30%.

B. Metamyelocytes can be seen in the peripheral blood.

C. Erythrocytosis is a predominant finding in the bone marrow.

D. Splenomegaly is a common finding.

E. Basophilia is a characteristic feature.

16. The following are statements regarding acute leukemia

A. Acute lymphoblastic leukemia is rare in children.

B. Auer rods are seen in acute myelobalstic leukemia (AML).

C. Gum bleeding is seen AML.

D. Radiation is a cause.

E. Hepatitis A is associated with T-cell leukemia.

17. Aetiology of lymphadenopathy include:

A. Leukaemia

B. Rhematoid arthritis

C. Cytomegalovirus infection

D. Acute respiratory failure

E. Disseminated intravascular haemolysis

18. The following are statements regarding non-Hodgkin lymphoma:

A. It is characterized histologically by Reed-Sternberg cells.

B. It is associated with alcohol induced pain.

C. Neoplastic lymphoid cells are of T or B cell origin.

D. HTLV-1 is associated with T cell lymphoma.

E. Extranodal involvement is common.

19. The following are statements regarding lymphomas

A.   It is a lymphoid malignancy involving the bone marrow.

B.   CNS lymphomas are common in HIV positive patients.

C.   Reed Sternberg cells are typical in Hodgkin lymphoma

D.   Epstein Barr virus is associated with Hodgkin lymphoma

E.   Generalised peripheral lymphadenopathy is common

20.   **The following are statements regarding multiple myeloma:**

A.   Serum uric acid level is high.

B.   M protein is seen on serum electrophoresis.

C.   Lytic lesion is seen on skull x-ray.

D.   An increased red blood cell synthesis is seen in the bone marrow.

E.   It commonly affects children.

21.   **Causes of paraproteinemia include:**

A.   Dengue fever

B.   Solitary plasmacytoma

C.   Waldenstrom macroglobulinaemia

D.   Systemic lupus erythematosis

E.   Heavy chain disease

22.   **Complications of multiple myeloma include:**

A.   Increased infection.

B.   Increased thrombosis.

C.   Renal stone formation.

D.   Cataract.

E.   Pathological fracture.

23.   **Complications of polycythemia vera include:**

   A.   Gum bleeding

   B.   Increased infection

   C.   Skin itchiness

   D.   Hypotension

   E.   Obesity

24.   **The following are statements regarding polycythemia rubra vera**

   A.   Arterial oxygen saturation is reduced

   B.   Serum uric acid is often raised

   C.   Neutral alkaline phosphatase is usually elevated

   D.   Leucocytosis is noted

   E.   Thrombocytosis is common

25.   **The following are statements regarding morphology of polycythemia vera**

A. Hemorrhages occur in about a third of patients.

B. Platelets may be dysfunctional in the disease.

C. The peripheral blood often shows increased basophils.

D. In bone marrow there is hyperplasia of erythroid, myloid, but not megakaryocytic forms.

E. Marrow fibrosis is present in 50% of patients.

26. **The following conditions are correctly matched to the inheritance method**

A. Thalassemia - autosomal dominant inheritance

B. Hemophilia A- X linked recessive

C. Spherocytosis - autosomal recessive inheritance

D. Eliptocytosis – autosomal dominant

E. Acute myeloid leukaemia - autosomal recessive

27. **The following are statements regarding genetic basis of hematological diseases:**

A. Sickle cell anaemia is due to point mutation of β globin gene.

B. t(8:14) translocation is found in Burkitt lymphoma.

C. Chronic myeloid leukemia is characterized by t(15;17) translocation

D. t(15;17) translocation is called Philadelphia chromosome

E. Fluorescent in-situ hybridization is a method of studying genetic abnormalities

28. **Causes of splenomegaly include:**

    A. Portal hypertension

    B. Malaria

    C. Hepatic failure

    D. Immune hemolytic anemia

    E. Idiopathic thrombocytopenia

29. **DiGeorge's syndrome is associated with**

    A. thymic aplasia

    B. failure of development of 3rd and 4th pharyngeal pouches

    C. hypercalcemia

    D. congenital cardiac abnormalities

    E. immunity against fungal infections

30. **The following are statements regarding sickle cell anemia**

    A. The sickling occurs because of a mutation in the hemoglobin gene

    B. The vaso-occlusive crisis is caused by sickle-shaped red blood cells that obstruct capillaries and restrict blood flow to an organ

    C. There is painful enlargement of the spleen due to Splenic sequestration crises

    D. Tachycardia and fatigue are presentation of Aplastic crises

E.   Cholelithiasis is a complication

5.1.b Questions with answers

1.   The following are statements regarding megaloblastic anaemia

T   A.   It is due to inhibition of DNA synthesis in red blood cell production

F   B.   Blood film shows microcytic red blood cells

T   C.   Alcohol abuse is one of the causes

T   D.   Present of nuclear hypersegmentation of neutrophils.

F   E.   Thrombocytosis is a finding.

2.   The following are statements regarding haemolytic anaemia

T   A.   In Microangiopathic Haemolytic Anemia (MAHA) the platelet count is decreased.

F   B.   Direct Coombs' test is positive in all of non immune cases.

F   C.   Conjugated bilirubin in the blood is elevated

F   D.   Sickle cell anaemia is associated with abnormality of RBC membrane.

T   E.   Blood smear shows elevated numbers of reticulocytes

3. **The following are statements regarding laboratory changes in anaemia:**

F   A.   Platelet count is increased in megaloblastic anaemia

F   B.   Total iron-binding capacity (TIBC) is low in iron deficiency anaemia

T   C.   There is low thyroid hormone level in some patients

T   D.   Serum lactate dehydrogenase (LDH) is elevated in haemolytic anaemia

F   E.   Blood smear show macrocytic changes in anaemia due to chronic blood loss

4. **The following are statements regarding thalassemia**

T   A.   It is an inherited autosomal recessive blood disorder

F   B.   Patient with thalassemia makes more hemoglobin but fewer circulating red blood cells than normal.

T   C.   Beta thalassemias are due to mutations in the HBB gene on chromosome 11.

F   D.   Iron supplements are useful in treatment

T   E.   Pneumonia is a complication

5. **The following are statements regarding Beta-thalassemias**

F   A.   Patient is usually presented at adolescence age with severe anemia

T   B.   In thalassemia mainor, only one of β globin alleles bears a mutation

T   C.   Severe bone deformities is a presentation in thalassemia major

T   D.   Cure is possible by bone marrow transplantation

T   E.   Affected patient requires regular lifelong blood transfusions.

6.   The following are statements regarding clotting disorders

T   A.   There is thrombocytopenia in laboratory evaluation.

T   B.   There is prolongation of PT and PTT.

T   C.   Fibrin split products are increased in the plasma

T   D.   DIC can be life threatening.

F   E.   The underlying disorder must not be treated simultaneously.

7.   Coagulation disorders include:

T   A.   Hemophilia (A, B).

T   B.   Von-Willebrand's disease.

T   C.   Vitamin-K deficiency.

F   D.   Henoch-Schonlein purpura.

F   E.   Idiopathic thrombocytopenic purpura (ITP).

8.   Causes of pancytopenia include:

T   A.   Multiple myeloma.

T   B.   Megaloblastic anemia.

T   C.   Aplastic anemia.

T   D.   Bone marrow infiltration.

F   E.   Sickle cell anemia.

9. Regarding Hemophilia

F   A.   Hemophilia A, accounts for about 80% of all cases, is a deficiency in clotting factor IX.

F   B.   The bleeding patterns and consequences of two types of hemophilia are different.

T   C.   Petechiae are characteristically absent.

F   D.   Cephalhematoma is one of characterstic features in infant females

F   E.   There is prolonged bleeding time.

10. Effects and complications of bone marrow failure include:

T   A.   Normochromic normocytic anemia.

T   B.   Thrombocytopenia.

T   C.   Increased susceptibility to infection.

T   D.   Neutrophilia.

F   E.   Presence of blast cells in the peripheral blood.

11. The following are statements regarding bone marrow failure

T   A.   Radiations is a cause

T   B.   Patient is susceptible easily to get infection

T   C.   Patient is anemic

F   D.   Bone marrow is hyperplastic

T   E.   Bone marrow aspiration is diagnostic

12. The following are statements regarding aplastic anemia

T   A.   Etiology is idiopathic, in more than half of cases.

F   B.   It increasingly appears that autoreactive B cells play an important role in pathogenesis.

T   C.   Bone marrow typically is markedly hypocellular

T   D.   In BM biopsy specimens; small foci of lymphcytes and plasma cells may be seen.

T   E.   Thrombocytopenia often presents as the appearance of petechiae and ecchymosis.

13. The following are statements regarding chronic myeloid leukemia:

F   A.   Philadelphia chromosome is absent in most of the cases.

F   B.   Neutrophil alkaline phosphatase score is increased.

T   C.   Normochromic normocytic anemia is usual.

T   D.   There is leucocytosis.

T   E.   Basophilia is common.

14. Characteristic features of acute leukaemias include :

T   A.   Children under 15 years most commonly affected in acute lymphoblastic leukemia(ALL)

F   B.   Gum hypertrophy is characteristic in acute lymphoblastic leukemia(ALL)

F   C.   Predominance of lymphoblasts in blood and bone marrow in acute myeloblastic leukemia(AML)

F   D.   Acid phosphatase diffuse positivity in leukaemic blasts in acute lymphoblastic leukemia(ALL)

T   E.   Remission rate is high in acute lymphoblastic leukemia(ALL)

15.   The following are statements regarding chronic myeloid leukemia

F   A.   The blast cells in peripheral blood smear are increased more than 30%.

T   B.   Metamyelocytes can be seen in the peripheral blood.

F   C.   Erythrocytosis is a predominant finding in the bone marrow.

T   D.   Splenomegaly is a common finding.

T   E.   Basophilia is a characteristic feature.

16.   The following are statements regarding acute leukemia

F   A.   Acute lymphoblastic leukemia is rare in children.

T   B.   Auer rods are seen in acute myelobalstic leukemia (AML).

T   C.   Gum bleeding is seen AML.

T   D.   Radiation is a cause.

F   E.   Hepatitis A is associated with T-cell leukemia.

17.   Aetiology of lymphadenopathy include:

T   A.   Leukaemia

T   B.   Rhematoid arthritis

T   C.   Cytomegalovirus infection

F   D.   Acute respiratory failure

F   E.   Disseminated intravascular haemolysis

18.   The following are statements regarding non-Hodgkin lymphoma:

F   A.   It is characterized histologically by Reed-Sternberg cells.

F   B.   It is associated with alcohol induced pain.

T   C.   Neoplastic lymphoid cells are of T or B cell origin.

T   D.   HTLV-1 is associated with T cell lymphoma.

T   E.   Extranodal involvement is common.

19.   The following are statements regarding lymphomas

F   A.   It is a lymphoid malignancy involving the bone marrow.

T   B.   CNS lymphomas are common in HIV positive patients.

F   C.   Reed Sternberg cells are typical in Hodgkin lymphoma

T   D.   Epstein Barr virus is associated with Hodgkin lymphoma

T   E.   Generalised peripheral lymphadenopathy is common

20.   The following are statements regarding multiple myeloma:

T   A.   Serum uric acid level is high.

T   B.   M protein is seen on serum electrophoresis.

T   C.   Lytic lesion is seen on skull x-ray.

F   D.   An increased red blood cell synthesis is seen in the bone marrow.

F   E.   It commonly affects children.

21.   Causes of paraproteinemia include:

F   A.   Dengue fever

T   B.   Solitary plasmacytoma

T   C.   Waldenstrom macroglobulinaemia

F   D.   Systemic lupus erythematosis

T   E.   Heavy chain disease

22.   Complications of multiple myeloma include:

T   A.   Increased infection.

F   B.   Increased thrombosis.

T   C.   Renal stone formation.

F   D.   Cataract.

T   E.   Pathological fracture.

23.   Complications of polycythemia vera include:

T   A.   Gum bleeding

T   B.   Increased infection

T   C.   Skin itchiness

F   D.   Hypotension

F   E.   Obesity

24.   The following are statements regarding polycythemia rubra vera

F   A.   Arterial oxygen saturation is reduced

T   B.   Serum uric acid is often raised

T   C.   Neutral alkaline phosphatase is usually elevated

T   D.   Leucocytosis is noted

T   E.   Thrombocytosis is common

25.   The following are statements regarding morphology of polycythemia vera

T   A.   Hemorrhages occur in about a third of patients.

T   B.   Platelets may be dysfunctional in the disease.

T   C.   The peripheral blood often shows increased basophils.

F   D.   In bone marrow there is hyperplasia of erythroid, myloid, but not megakaryocytic forms.

F   E.   Marrow fibrosis is present in 50% of patients.

26. The following conditions are correctly matched to the inheritance method

F   A.   Thalassemia - autosomal dominant inheritance

T   B.   Hemophilia A- X linked recessive

F   C.   Spherocytosis - autosomal recessive inheritance

T   D.   Eliptocytosis – autosomal dominant

F   E.   Acute myeloid leukaemia - autosomal recessive

27. The following are statements regarding genetic basis of hematological diseases:

F   A.   Sickle cell anaemia is due to point mutation of β globin gene.

T   B.   t(8:14) translocation is found in Burkitt lymphoma.

T   C.   Chronic myeloid leukemia is characterized by t(15;17) translocation

T   D.   t(15;17) translocation is called Philadelphia chromosome

T   E.   Fluorescent in-situ hybridization is a method of studying genetic abnormalities

28. Causes of splenomegaly include:

T   A.   Portal hypertension

T   B.   Malaria

F   C.   Hepatic failure

T   D.   Immune hemolytic anemia

T   E.   Idiopathic thrombocytopenia

29.   DiGeorge's syndrome is associated with

T   A.   thymic aplasia

T   B.   failure of development of 3rd and 4th pharyngeal pouches

F   C.   hypercalcemia

T   D.   congenital cardiac abnormalities

F   E.   immunity against fungal infections

30.   The following are statements regarding sickle cell anemia

T   A.   The sickling occurs because of a mutation in the hemoglobin gene

T   B.   The vaso-occlusive crisis is caused by sickle-shaped red blood cells that obstruct capillaries and restrict blood flow to an organ

T   C.   There is painful enlargement of the spleen due to Splenic sequestration crises

T   D.   Tachycardia and fatigue are presentation of Aplastic crises

T   E.   Cholelithiasis is a complication

5.2 IMMUNOLOGY

5.2.a Questions without answers

1. **The following are statements regarding the organization of the immune system:**

A.   Thymus is a primary lymphoid organ.

B.   Maturation of lymphocytes occurs in secondary lymphoid organs.

C.   Adaptive immunity is less specific than the innate immunity.

D.   Tolerance to self-antigen is generated only in the innate immune response.

E.   Naïve lymphocytes are mature cells which remain in the bone marrow.

2. **The following are statements regarding innate immunity:**

A.   Mucosal epithelia form the physical barrier.

B.   Antibody production is enhanced with successive exposure to a particular antigen.

C.   The cellular component consists of the lymphocytes and their products.

D.   There is non-reactivity to self-antigen.

E.   Memory cells are generated following antigen stimulation.

3.   **The following are statements regarding cells and tissues of the immune system:**

A.   Bone marrow is a secondary lymphoid organ where responses to foreign antigens are stimulated.

B.   Natural killer cells recognize and kill virus-infected and tumor cells.

C.   Only B cells express antigen receptors which are required in antigen recognition.

D.   Follicular dendritic cells act as antigen presenting cells in the lymph nodes.

E.   Cytotoxic T cells have CD4+ surface molecules.

4.   **The following are statements regarding lymphocytes:**

A.   B cells attain full maturation in the bone marrow.

B.   Helper T cells carry CD8+ molecules on the surface.

C.   Naïve cells are mature lymphocytes which have encountered several antigens.

D.   Natural killer cells are lymphocytes involved in antibody-dependent cell cytotoxicity.

E.   Lymphocytes are the main cells involved in innate immunity.

5. **Haptens**

    A. are substances with low molecular weight.

    B. induce immune response only when coupled to a carrier molecule.

    C. are capable of binding to an antibody.

    D. induce the production of only IgM antibody.

    E. prolong the retention of an immunogen when injected.

6. **T-dependent antigens**

    A. have polymeric structure.

    B. are usually polysaccharides.

    C. are more readily degraded by phagocytes.

    D. are polyclonal activators of B cells.

    E. stimulate the production of antibodies without T cell help.

7. **The following are statements regarding the general features of antibodies:**

    A. Each antibody molecule is composed of 4 identical light and 4 heavy chains.

    B. Kappa ($\varkappa$) & lambda (λ) are examples of heavy chains.

    C. Some antibodies are present in cytoplasmic membrane-bound compartments of B-cells.

    D. J chain is only found in IgM.

E.   Complementarity Determining Regions (CDRs) from both the light and heavy chains form the antigen binding site.

8.   **Immunoglobulin E (IgE)**

   A.   binds to the surface of mast cells.

   B.   is always in the form of dimer.

   C.   is responsible for the symptoms of atopic allergy.

   D.   level is raised in helminthic infections.

   E.   is found in high concentration in serum.

9.   **Immunoglobulin M (IgM)**

   A.   is in the form of a pentamer.

   B.   readily passes through the placenta.

   C.   is a excellent activator of complements.

   D.   is present as a monomer on the surface of B cells.

   E.   plays an important role in immediate hypersensitivity reactions.

10.   **Complement proteins**

   A.   are plasma proteins which are normally active.

   B.   are heat-stable.

   C.   are antigen-specific.

D. C6 to C9 are devoid of proteolytic activity.

E. are only activated in the presence of IgM.

11. **The following are statements regarding classical pathway of complement activation:**

A. C1q binds to the Fc portion of the antibody that has bound antigen.

B. C4bC2b (C4b2b) is the C3 convertase of the classical complement pathway.

C. Only the classical pathway produces C5 convertase.

D. Cleavage of C4 is the initiation of the late steps of complement activation.

E. C4a stimulates inflammatory response.

12. **Major histocompatibility complex genes**

A. are found on the short arm of chromosome 6.

B. are highly polymorphic.

C. of the Class I code for HLA-DP, HLA-DQ and HLA-DR.

D. of the Class II code for HLA-A, HLA-B and HLA-C.

E. of the Class III code for complement components.

13. **MHC (major histocompatibility complex) Class I molecules**

A.   contain two polypeptide chains, α and β_2-microglobulin.

B.   have peptide binding cleft which is formed by α_1 and α_2.

C.   are found on the surface of red blood cells.

D.   contain the binding site for T cell co-receptor CD4.

E.   include HLA-A, HLA-B and HLA-C.

14.   **The following are statements regarding cardinal features of the adaptive immunity:**

A.   Parts of antigens that are specifically recognized by lymphocytes are called epitopes.

B.   Each exposure to an antigen expands clone of lymphocytes specific for the particular antigen.

C.   Memory T cells produce lower affinity antibodies which bind antigens.

D.   Cell-mediated immunity responds to extracellular organisms.

E.   All normal immune responses wane with time after antigen stimulation.

15.   **Compared to primary immune response, secondary immune response to T-dependent antigens:**

A.   has longer lag phase.

B.   consists of almost entirely of IgM with very little IgG.

C.   produces antibody with much lower affinity.

D.   results in the production of antibody in higher titres.

E.   produces antibody which persists for a longer period.

16.   Phases of the humoral immune response include

A.   recognition of antigens via the surface immunoglobulin receptors on B cells.

B.   proliferation and differentiation of specific B cell clones.

C.   production of IgM and other isotypes.

D.   an isotype switch and affinity maturation.

E.   development of memory cells only from B cells.

17.   The following are statements regarding cell-mediated cytotoxicity:

A.   It is an essential defense against the extracellular pathogens.

B.   NK cells are involved in killing of target cells without the MHC Class I molecules.

C.   Cytotoxicity occurs by direct cellular interaction via the surface molecules.

D.   It does not involve the role of the cytokines.

E.   Formation of polyperforin channels on cell membrane and influx of granzymes leads to death of target cells.

18.   Cytotoxic lymphocytes / cytotoxic T cells (CTLs/Tc)

A. recognize antigens that are presented on MHC Class II.

B. play an important role in the elimination of extracellular pathogens.

C. antagonize the action of NK cells in the destruction of viral-infected cells.

D. kill target cells through indirect signaling via the cytokines.

E. release granzymes upon recognition of target cells.

19. Cytokines

A. are small proteins that act only in the paracrine manner.

B. act by binding to specific receptors at the cell membrane.

C. usually act alone.

D. are involved in the T cell proliferation.

E. include the interleukins and colony stimulating factors.

20. The following are pairs of types of hypersensitivity and their immune mechanisms:

A. Type I : Complements are activated via the classical pathway.

B. Type I : It is also called antibody-dependent cell cytotoxicity.

C. Type II : The target cells are destroyed only via complement activated lysis.

D.   Type III   :   In antigen excess, the immune complexes are deposited on the glomerular basement membrane.

E.   Type IV   :   There is a chronic stimulation of T cells and release of cytokines.

21. **A 35-year-old man had a bee sting while clearing his backyard. A few minutes later, his face became swollen. The following are statements regarding the case:**

A.   This is an example of Type III hypersensitivity reaction.

B.   This condition is more common in atopic individuals.

C.   Cross-linking of the Fcε receptors by the allergen causes degranulation of mast cells.

D.   Both preformed and newly synthesized chemical mediators are released.

E.   If left untreated, the condition can result in anaphylactic shock.

22. **The following are statements regarding hypersensitivity type 1:**

A.   Mast cells and basophils form the major cellular component.

B.   There is activation of complements via the classical pathways.

C.   The reaction occurs at least few days after an exposure to an allergen.

D.   Histamine is an example of newly synthesized chemical

mediators.

E.   Sodium cromoglycate is one of the drugs used in the treatment.

23.   **Hemolytic disease of newborn due to Rhesus incompatibility**

A.   is an example of hypersensitivity type III.

B.   is more commonly seen in the first born baby.

C.   occurs when RhD positive mother carrying RhD negative fetus.

D.   may result in hydrops fetalis.

E.   can be prevented by injecting anti-D immediately postpartum.

24.   **The following are statements regarding mechanisms of Type III hypersensitivity:**

A.   It is due to persistence and deposition of immune complexes in tissues.

B.   The Arthus reaction occurs in antigen excess.

C.   In serum sickness, there is marked edema at the antigen injection site.

D.   The immune complexes act on the mast cells which release the vasoactive amines.

E.   The inflammation is due to the lysosomal enzymes released by the polymorphs.

25. **The following are statements regarding hypersensitivity type IV:**

    A.   It is a cell-mediated immunity.

    B.   Langerhans cells are the main antigen presenting cells in contact hypersensitivity.

    C.   Cytokines are produced by antigen-specific T cells.

    D.   Granuloma formation is one of its characteristic features.

    E.   Myasthenia gravis is an example.

26. **A 27-year-old lady complains of swelling of the neck associated with "big eyes" for a few months. The attending doctor suspects an autoimmune disease. The following statements are true regarding the case:**

    A.   Graves' disease can be considered as a differential diagnosis.

    B.   It is a non-organ-specific autoimmune disease.

    C.   Antibody may be detected against the thyroid cells.

    D.   Type III hypersensitivity reactions may play a role in the immunopathology.

    E.   Antibody produced usually destroys the thyroid cells.

27. **A 35-year-old lady presents with history of morning stiffness of the fingers for one month. The attending doctor suspects an autoimmune disease. The following statements are true regarding this case:**

A. Rheumatoid arthritis can be considered as a differential diagnosis.

B. It is likely to an organ-specific autoimmune disease.

C. Type II hypersensitivity reactions may play a role in the immunopathology.

D. It may be associated with gastric autoimmunity.

E. She can be treated with anti-inflammatory drugs.

28. **Tumor cells evade the immune system by the following mechanisms:**

A. Tumor cells share antigens with the normal tissue from which they arise.

B. Viruses (eg EBV) may inhibit proteasome processing of antigen.

C. Some tumors reduce the MHC expression and impair the NK activity.

D. Tumor cells express high levels of co-stimulatory molecules eg B7.

E. Tumor cells do not always activate the innate immune system.

29. **The following are pairs of primary immunodeficiency and its immunological defects:**

A. Chronic granulomatous disease   :   Defective killing by phagocytes

B. Hereditary angioedema   :   Complement C1

deficiency

C. Chediak-Higashi syndrome : Primary B cell deficiency

D. Bruton's disease : Primary T cell deficiency

E. Selective IgA deficiency : Failure in the terminal differentiation of B cells.

30. Di George syndrome

A. is a congenital defect of organs derived from the 3rd and 4th pharyngeal pouches.

B. presents with abnormal facies, low set ears and micrognathia.

C. is susceptible to viral and fungal infections.

D. is characterized by a complete absence of B cell function.

E. is treated with thymus graft.

5.2.b Questions with answers

1. **The following are statements regarding the organization of the immune system:**

T   A.   Thymus is a primary lymphoid organ.

F   B.   Maturation of lymphocytes occurs in secondary lymphoid organs.

F   C.   Adaptive immunity is less specific than the innate immunity.

F   D.   Tolerance to self-antigen is generated only in the innate immune response.

F   E.   Naïve lymphocytes are mature cells which remain in the bone marrow.

2. **The following are statements regarding innate immunity:**

T   A.   Mucosal epithelia form the physical barrier.

F   B.   Antibody production is enhanced with successive exposure to a particular antigen.

F   C.   The cellular component consists of the lymphocytes and their products.

T   D.   There is non-reactivity to self-antigen.

F   E.   Memory cells are generated following antigen stimulation.

3. The following are statements regarding cells and tissues of the immune system:

F A. Bone marrow is a secondary lymphoid organ where responses to foreign antigens are stimulated.

T B. Natural killer cells recognize and kill virus-infected and tumor cells.

F C. Only B cells express antigen receptors which are required in antigen recognition.

T D. Follicular dendritic cells act as antigen presenting cells in the lymph nodes.

F E. Cytotoxic T cells have CD4+ surface molecules.

4. The following are statements regarding lymphocytes:

T A. B cells attain full maturation in the bone marrow.

F B. Helper T cells carry CD8+ molecules on the surface.

F C. Naïve cells are mature lymphocytes which have encountered several antigens.

T D. Natural killer cells are lymphocytes involved in antibody-dependent cell cytotoxicity.

F E. Lymphocytes are the main cells involved in innate immunity.

5. Haptens

T A. are substances with low molecular weight.

T   B.   induce immune response only when coupled to a carrier molecule.

T   C.   are capable of binding to an antibody.

F   D.   induce the production of only IgM antibody.

F   E.   prolong the retention of an immunogen when injected.

6.   T-dependent antigens

F   A.   have polymeric structure.

F   B.   are usually polysaccharides.

T   C.   are more readily degraded by phagocytes.

F   D.   are polyclonal activators of B cells.

F   E.   stimulate the production of antibodies without T cell help.

7.   The following are statements regarding the general features of antibodies:

F   A.   Each antibody molecule is composed of 4 identical light and 4 heavy chains.

F   B.   Kappa ($\varkappa$) & lambda (λ) are examples of heavy chains.

T   C.   Some antibodies are present in cytoplasmic membrane-bound compartments of B-cells.

F   D.   J chain is only found in IgM.

T   E.   Complementarity Determining Regions (CDRs) from both the light and heavy chains form the antigen binding site.

8. Immunoglobulin E (IgE)

T   A.   binds to the surface of mast cells.

F   B.   is always in the form of dimer.

T   C.   is responsible for the symptoms of atopic allergy.

T   D.   level is raised in helminthic infections.

F   E.   is found in high concentration in serum.

9. Immunoglobulin M (IgM)

T   A.   is in the form of a pentamer.

F   B.   readily passes through the placenta.

T   C.   is a excellent activator of complements.

T   D.   is present as a monomer on the surface of B cells.

F   E.   plays an important role in immediate hypersensitivity reactions.

10. Complement proteins

F   A.   are plasma proteins which are normally active.

F   B.   are heat-stable.

F   C.   are antigen-specific.

T   D.   C6 to C9 are devoid of proteolytic activity.

F   E.   are only activated in the presence of IgM.

11. **The following are statements regarding classical pathway of complement activation:**

T   A.   C1q binds to the Fc portion of the antibody that has bound antigen.

T   B.   C4bC2b (C4b2b) is the C3 convertase of the classical complement pathway.

F   C.   Only the classical pathway produces C5 convertase.

F   D.   Cleavage of C4 is the initiation of the late steps of complement activation.

T   E.   C4a stimulates inflammatory response.

12. **Major histocompatibility complex genes**

T   A.   are found on the short arm of chromosome 6.

T   B.   are highly polymorphic.

F   C.   of the Class I code for HLA-DP, HLA-DQ and HLA-DR.

F   D.   of the Class II code for HLA-A, HLA-B and HLA-C.

T   E.   of the Class III code for complement components.

13. **MHC (major histocompatibility complex) Class I molecules**

T   A.   contain two polypeptide chains, α and β_2-microglobulin.

T   B.   have peptide binding cleft which is formed by α_1 and α_2.

F   C.   are found on the surface of red blood cells.

F   D.   contain the binding site for T cell co-receptor CD4.

T   E.   include HLA-A, HLA-B and HLA-C.

14.   The following are statements regarding cardinal features of the adaptive immunity:

T   A.   Parts of antigens that are specifically recognized by lymphocytes are called epitopes.

T   B.   Each exposure to an antigen expands clone of lymphocytes specific for the particular antigen.

F   C.   Memory T cells produce lower affinity antibodies which bind antigens.

F   D.   Cell-mediated immunity responds to extracellular organisms.

T   E.   All normal immune responses wane with time after antigen stimulation.

15.   Compared to primary immune response, secondary immune response to T-dependent antigens:

F   A.   has longer lag phase.

F   B.   consists of almost entirely of IgM with very little IgG.

F   C.   produces antibody with much lower affinity.

T   D.   results in the production of antibody in higher titres.

T   E.   produces antibody which persists for a longer period.

16.   Phases of the humoral immune response include

T   A.   recognition of antigens via the surface immunoglobulin receptors on B cells.

T   B.   proliferation and differentiation of specific B cell clones.

T   C.   production of IgM and other isotypes.

T   D.   an isotype switch and affinity maturation.

F   E.   development of memory cells only from B cells.

17. The following are statements regarding cell-mediated cytotoxicity:

F   A.   It is an essential defense against the extracellular pathogens.

T   B.   NK cells are involved in killing of target cells without the MHC Class I molecules.

T   C.   Cytotoxicity occurs by direct cellular interaction via the surface molecules.

F   D.   It does not involve the role of the cytokines.

T   E.   Formation of polyperforin channels on cell membrane and influx of granzymes leads to death of target cells.

18. Cytotoxic lymphocytes / cytotoxic T cells (CTLs/Tc)

F   A.   recognize antigens that are presented on MHC Class II.

F   B.   play an important role in the elimination of extracellular pathogens.

F   C.   antagonize the action of NK cells in the destruction of viral-infected cells.

T   D.   kill target cells through indirect signaling via the cytokines.

T   E.   release granzymes upon recognition of target cells.

19.   Cytokines

F   A.   are small proteins that act only in the paracrine manner.

T   B.   act by binding to specific receptors at the cell membrane.

F   C.   usually act alone.

T   D.   are involved in the T cell proliferation.

T   E.   include the interleukins and colony stimulating factors.

20.   The following are pairs of types of hypersensitivity and their immune mechanisms:

F   A.   Type I   :   Complements are activated via the classical pathway.

F   B.   Type I   :   It is also called antibody-dependent cell cytotoxicity.

F   C.   Type II   :   The target cells are destroyed only via complement activated lysis.

T   D.   Type III   :   In antigen excess, the immune complexes are deposited on the glomerular basement membrane.

T   E.   Type IV   :   There is a chronic stimulation of T cells and release of cytokines.

21. **A 35-year-old man had a bee sting while clearing his backyard. A few minutes later, his face became swollen. The following are statements regarding the case:**

F   A.   This is an example of Type III hypersensitivity reaction.

T   B.   This condition is more common in atopic individuals.

T   C.   Cross-linking of the Fcε receptors by the allergen causes degranulation of mast cells.

T   D.   Both preformed and newly synthesized chemical mediators are released.

T   E.   If left untreated, the condition can result in anaphylactic shock.

22. **The following are statements regarding hypersensitivity type 1:**

T   A.   Mast cells and basophils form the major cellular component.

F   B.   There is activation of complements via the classical pathways.

F   C.   The reaction occurs at least few days after an exposure to an allergen.

F   D.   Histamine is an example of newly synthesized chemical mediators.

T   E.   Sodium cromoglycate is one of the drugs used in the treatment.

23. **Hemolytic disease of newborn due to Rhesus incompatibility**

F   A.   is an example of hypersensitivity type III.

F   B.   is more commonly seen in the first born baby.

F   C.   occurs when RhD positive mother carrying RhD negative fetus.

T   D.   may result in hydrops fetalis.

T   E.   can be prevented by injecting anti-D immediately postpartum.

24. **The following are statements regarding mechanisms of Type III hypersensitivity:**

T   A.   It is due to persistence and deposition of immune complexes in tissues.

F   B.   The Arthus reaction occurs in antigen excess.

F   C.   In serum sickness, there is marked edema at the antigen injection site.

T   D.   The immune complexes act on the mast cells which release the vasoactive amines.

T   E.   The inflammation is due to the lysosomal enzymes released by the polymorphs.

25. **The following are statements regarding hypersensitivity type IV:**

T   A.   It is a cell-mediated immunity.

F   B.   Langerhans cells are the main antigen presenting cells in contact hypersensitivity.

T   C.   Cytokines are produced by antigen-specific T cells.

T   D.   Granuloma formation is one of its characteristic features.

F   E.   Myasthenia gravis is an example.

26.   **A 27-year-old lady complains of swelling of the neck associated with "big eyes" for a few months. The attending doctor suspects an autoimmune disease. The following statements are true regarding the case:**

T   A.   Graves' disease can be considered as a differential diagnosis.

F   B.   It is a non-organ-specific autoimmune disease.

F   C.   Antibody may be detected against the thyroid cells.

F   D.   Type III hypersensitivity reactions may play a role in the immunopathology.

F   E.   Antibody produced usually destroys the thyroid cells.

27.   **A 35-year-old lady presents with history of morning stiffness of the fingers for one month. The attending doctor suspects an autoimmune disease. The following statements are true regarding this case:**

T   A.   Rheumatoid arthritis can be considered as a differential diagnosis.

F   B.   It is likely to an organ-specific autoimmune disease.

F   C.   Type II hypersensitivity reactions may play a role in the immunopathology.

F   D.   It may be associated with gastric autoimmunity.

T   E.   She can be treated with anti-inflammatory drugs.

28. Tumor cells evade the immune system by the following mechanisms:

T   A.   Tumor cells share antigens with the normal tissue from which they arise.

T   B.   Viruses (eg EBV) may inhibit proteasome processing of antigen.

F   C.   Some tumors reduce the MHC expression and impair the NK activity.

F   D.   Tumor cells express high levels of co-stimulatory molecules eg B7.

F   E.   Tumor cells do not always activate the innate immune system.

29. The following are pairs of primary immunodeficiency and its immunological defects:

T   A.   Chronic granulomatous disease   :   Defective killing by phagocytes

F   B.   Hereditary angioedema   :   Complement C1 deficiency

F   C.   Chediak-Higashi syndrome   :   Primary B cell deficiency

F   D.   Bruton's disease   :   Primary T cell deficiency

T   E.   Selective IgA deficiency   :   Failure in the terminal differentiation of B cells.

30. Di George syndrome

T   A.   is a congenital defect of organs derived from the 3rd and 4th pharyngeal pouches.

T   B.   presents with abnormal facies, low set ears and micrognathia.

T   C.   is susceptible to viral and fungal infections.

F   D.   is characterized by a complete absence of B cell function.

T   E.   is treated with thymus graft.

6 GASTROINTESTINAL SYSTEM

6.1 Pathology of Gastrointestinal System

6.1.a Questions without answers

1.   The following are statements regarding nasopharyngeal carcinoma:

A.   It is strongly associated with HPV virus infection.

B.   Cervical lymphadenopathy is the initial presentation in many patients.

C.   Trismus is a clinical presentation

D.   It is vastly more common in certain regions of East Asia

E.   lymph node biopsy is diagnostic.

2.   The following are statements regarding Barrett's esophagus:

A.   It refers to dysplasia in the cells of the lower portion of the esophagus

B.   It is precancerous lesion of esophageal adenocarcinoma

C.   Reflux esophagitis is the main cause

D.   It is marked by the presence of columnar epithelia in the lower esophagus

E.   Both macroscopic and microscopic positive findings are required to make a diagnosis.

3.   **Morphological features of reflux oesophagitis include**

A.   Hperaemia of the mucosa and focal hemorrhage in gross specomen.

B.   Epithelial hyperplasia.

C.   Infiltration of neutrophils

D.   Intraepithelial eosinophils

E.   Granuloma

4.   **The following are statements regarding hiatus hernia**

A.   Sliding type is more common than rolling type

B.   Rolling type predisposes to reflux oesophagitis

C.   It occurs due to weakness of the central tendon of diaphragm

D.   It is more common in infants compared to adults

E.   Obstruction is a complication of the sliding type

5. **The following are statements regarding achalasia**

   A.   There is decrease lower eosphageal sphincter tone.

   B.   The oesophagus has increased peristalsis

   C.   Chagas disease is a cause

   D.   Complications include aspiration pneumonia

   E.   The affected patients are mostly above 60 years of age

6. **The following are statements regarding oesophageal varices**

   A.   It involves the anastomosis of left gastric vein and azygous vein

   B.   Liver cirrhosis is one of the causes

   C.   It predisposes to squamous cell carcinoma of upper oesophagus

   D.   The mucosa of the involved segment bulges outward

   E.   If bleeding occurs, the mortality rate is high.

7. **The following are statements regarding carcinoma of esophagus:**

   A.   Squamous cell carcinoma arises commonly at the lower end of esophagus.

   B.   Barrett's esophagus is metaplastic squamous eptihelium.

   C.   Tracheo-esophageal fistula is a complication.

   D.   Clinically presents with dysphagia.

   E.   Betel chewing is a risk factor.

8. **The following are statements regarding peptic ulcers**

    A. Helicobacter pylori is an important cause.

    B. Commonly affects the first part of duodenum

    C. Benign ulcers have overhanging shaggy margins.

    D. Perforation is a complication

    E. Usually associated with hyperaciditiy.

9. **The following are statements regarding stomach cancer**

    A. It is mostly caused by Helicobacter pylori infection.

    B. Eating of salted fish is a risk factor

    C. There is female predominance in its incidence as up to three females are affected for every male

    D. Prognosis is poor

    E. Majority of gastric malignancies are lymphomas

10. **The following are statements regarding malabsorption:**

    A. Steatorrhoea is a common clinical symptom.

    B. Weight gain and increased appetite are common.

    C. Coeliac disease is treated by broad spectrum antibiotic

    D. Villous atrophy is a classical histological feature.

    E. Tropical sprue is associated with risk of intestinal lymphoma.

11. **The following are statements regarding intestinal obstruction:**

   A.   Internal or external hernia is a major cause of mechanical obstruction.

   B.   Paralytic ileus is a cause of pseudo-obstruction.

   C.   Adhesions may develop between bowel segments after surgical procedures.

   D.   Intussusception always occurs without apparent anatomic basis.

   E.   Volvulus refers to twisting of a loop of bowel or other structure as the ovary.

12. **Crohn's disease in comparison with ulcerative colitis "UC**

   A.   Terminal ileum involvement is common in UC while it is rare in Crohn's.

   B.   Colon is usually involved in Crohn's while it always involved in UC.

   C.   Involvement around the anus is common in Crohn's while it is rare in UC

   D.   Stenosis is common in Crohn's while it is rare in UC

   E.   Granulomas on biopsy is seen in Crohn's while it is not found in UC.

13. **Symptoms of acute cholecystitis include:**

   A.   The main symptom is pain in the upper right side or upper middle of the abdomen

   B.   The pain can spreads to the back or below the right shoulder blade

C.   Hypertention

D.   Jaundice

E.   Nausea and vomiting

14.   Clinical manifestations of cirrhosis include:

A.   Jaundice.

B.   Tender hepatomegaly.

C.   Ascites.

D.   Caput medusa.

E.   Portal hypertension.

15.   Conditions found in liver failure include:

A.   Ascitis.

B.   Hyperplasia of the gonads.

C.   Hypoalbuminemia.

D.   Splenomegaly.

E.   Spider naevi.

16.   Regarding Hepatitis A infection

A.   It usually spread by the fecal-oral route

B.   The incubation period is between two and six weeks and the average incubation period is 28 days.

C.   It is a self-limited disease in majority of cases

D.   The disease can be prevented by vaccination

E.   Fatigue is a presentation

17.   **The following are statements regarding hepatitis:**

A.   Ground glass hepatocytes are characteristic of hepatitis B.

B.   Mallory hyaline is seen in alcoholic hepatitis.

C.   Fibrosis is a hall mark of reversible tissue damage in hepatitis A.

D.   Councilman body is commonly seen in acute hepatitis.

E.   Bridging fibrosis is uncommon in chronic active hepatitis.

18.   **The following are statements regarding hepatocellular carcinoma**

A.   Hepatitis B virus is implicated in the pathogenesis

B.   The prognosis is good.

C.   The liver is cirrhotic in many of the patients

D.   Fibrolamellar type tends to occur in the older age group

E.   Invasion of vascular channels is a feature

19.   **Most common causes of acute pancreatitis include:**

A.   Alcohol

B.   Smoking

C.   Gallstones

D.   Hypocalcemia

E.   Malignancy

20.   **The following are statements regarding chronic pancreatitis**

A.   Steatorrhea is a presentation

B.   It can present as episodes of acute inflammation in a previously injured pancreas.

C.   Serum amylase is always elevated

D.   In developed countries, the most common cause is alcohol.

E.   Diabetes is a common complication

6.1.b Questions with answers

1. The following are statements regarding nasopharyngeal carcinoma:

F   A.   It is strongly associated with HPV virus infection.

T   B.   Cervical lymphadenopathy is the initial presentation in many patients.

T   C.   Trismus is a clinical presentation

T   D.   It is vastly more common in certain regions of East Asia

T   E.   lymph node biopsy is diagnostic.

2. The following are statements regarding Barrett's esophagus:

F   A.   It refers to dysplasia in the cells of the lower portion of the esophagus

T   B.   It is precancerous lesion of esophageal adenocarcinoma

T   C.   Reflux esophagitis is the main cause

T   D.   It is marked by the presence of columnar epithelia in the lower esophagus

T   E.   Both macroscopic and microscopic positive findings are required to make a diagnosis.

3.   Morphological features of reflux oesophagitis include

T   A.   Hperaemia of the mucosa and focal hemorrhage in gross specomen.

T   B.   Epithelial hyperplasia.

T   C.   Infiltration of neutrophils

T   D.   Intraepithelial eosinophils

F   E.   Granuloma

4.   The following are statements regarding hiatus hernia

T   A.   Sliding type is more common than rolling type

F   B.   Rolling type predisposes to reflux oesophagitis

F   C.   It occurs due to weakness of the central tendon of diaphragm

F   D.   It is more common in infants compared to adults

F   E.   Obstruction is a complication of the sliding type

5.   The following are statements regarding achalasia

F   A.   There is decrease lower eosphageal sphincter tone.

F   B.   The oesophagus has increased peristalsis

T   C.   Chagas disease is a cause

T   D.   Complications include aspiration pneumonia

F   E.   The affected patients are mostly above 60 years of age

6.   The following are statements regarding oesophageal varices

T   A.   It involves the anastomosis of left gastric vein and azygous vein

T   B.   Liver cirrhosis is one of the causes

F   C.   It predisposes to squamous cell carcinoma of upper oesophagus

T   D.   The mucosa of the involved segment bulges outward

T   E.   If bleeding occurs, the mortality rate is high.

7.   The following are statements regarding carcinoma of esophagus:

F   A.   Squamous cell carcinoma arises commonly at the lower end of esophagus.

F   B.   Barrett's esophagus is metaplastic squamous eptihelium.

T   C.   Tracheo-esophageal fistula is a complication.

T   D.   Clinically presents with dysphagia.

T   E.   Betel chewing is a risk factor.

8.   The following are statements regarding peptic ulcers

T   A.   Helicobacter pylori is an important cause.

T   B.   Commonly affects the first part of duodenum

F   C.   Benign ulcers have overhanging shaggy margins.

T   D.   Perforation is a complication

T   E.   Usually associated with hyperaciditiy.

9. The following are statements regarding stomach cancer

T   A.   It is mostly caused by Helicobacter pylori infection.

T   B.   Eating of salted fish is a risk factor

F   C.   There is female predominance in its incidence as up to three females are affected for every male

T   D.   Prognosis is poor

F   E.   Majority of gastric malignancies are lymphomas

10. The following are statements regarding malabsorption:

T   A.   Steatorrhoea is a common clinical symptom.

F   B.   Weight gain and increased appetite are common.

F   C.   Coeliac disease is treated by broad spectrum antibiotic

T   D.   Villous atrophy is a classical histological feature.

F   E.   Tropical sprue is associated with risk of intestinal lymphoma.

11. The following are statements regarding intestinal obstruction:

T   A.   Internal or external hernia is a major cause of mechanical obstruction.

T   B.   Paralytic ileus is a cause of pseudo-obstruction.

T   C.   Adhesions may develop between bowel segments after surgical procedures.

F   D.   Intussusception always occurs without apparent anatomic basis.

T   E.   Volvulus refers to twisting of a loop of bowel or other structure as the ovary.

12. Crohn's disease in comparison with ulcerative colitis "UC

F   A.   Terminal ileum involvement is common in UC while it is rare in Crohn's.

T   B.   Colon is usually involved in Crohn's while it always involved in UC.

T   C.   Involvement around the anus is common in Crohn's while it is rare in UC

T   D.   Stenosis is common in Crohn's while it is rare in UC

T   E.   Granulomas on biopsy is seen in Crohn's while it is not found in UC.

13. Symptoms of acute cholecystitis include:

T   A.   The main symptom is pain in the upper right side or upper middle of the abdomen

T   B.   The pain can spreads to the back or below the right shoulder blade

F   C.   Hypertention

T   D.   Jaundice

T   E.   Nausea and vomiting

14. Clinical manifestations of cirrhosis include:

T   A.   Jaundice.

F   B.   Tender hepatomegaly.

T   C.   Ascites.

T   D.   Caput medusa.

T   E.   Portal hypertension.

15.   Conditions found in liver failure include:

T   A.   Ascitis.

F   B.   Hyperplasia of the gonads.

T   C.   Hypoalbuminemia.

T   D.   Splenomegaly.

T   E.   Spider naevi.

16.   Regarding Hepatitis A infection

T   A.   It usually spread by the fecal-oral route

T   B.   The incubation period is between two and six weeks and the average incubation period is 28 days.

T   C.   It is a self-limited disease in majority of cases

T   D.   The disease can be prevented by vaccination

T   E.   Fatigue is a presentation

17.   The following are statements regarding hepatitis:

T   A.   Ground glass hepatocytes are characteristic of hepatitis B.

T   B.   Mallory hyaline is seen in alcoholic hepatitis.

F   C.   Fibrosis is a hall mark of reversible tissue damage in hepatitis A.

T   D.   Councilman body is commonly seen in acute hepatitis.

F   E.   Bridging fibrosis is uncommon in chronic active hepatitis.

18.   The following are statements regarding hepatocellular carcinoma

T   A.   Hepatitis B virus is implicated in the pathogenesis

F   B.   The prognosis is good.

T   C.   The liver is cirrhotic in many of the patients

F   D.   Fibrolamellar type tends to occur in the older age group

T   E.   Invasion of vascular channels is a feature

19.   Most common causes of acute pancreatitis include:

T   A.   Alcohol

T   B.   Smoking

T   C.   Gallstones

F   D.   Hypocalcemia

T   E.   Malignancy

20.   The following are statements regarding chronic pancreatitis

T   A.   Steatorrhea is a presentation

T   B.   It can present as episodes of acute inflammation in a previously injured pancreas.

F   C.   Serum amylase is always elevated

T   D.   In developed countries, the most common cause is alcohol.

T   E.   Diabetes is a common complication

6.2 Microbiology of Gastrointestinal System

6.2.a Questions without answers

1. **The following are statements regarding cholera:**

   A. It is only caused by *Vibrio cholerae* serotype O1.

   B. The causative organism usually invades into the bloodstream.

   C. It is due to the heat-labile enterotoxin released by the causative organism.

   D. Profuse watery diarrhea and abdominal cramps are the common clinical manifestations.

   E. Treatment consists of fluid and electrolyte replacement and doxycycline.

2. **The following are statements regarding typhoid fever:**

   A. It is caused by *Salmonella paratyphi* A, B and C.

   B. Its causative organism multiplies in intestinal lymphoid tissue and excreted in stools.

   C. Fever and hepatosplenomegaly are the common clinical manifestations.

   D. Stool culture is usually positive in first week of the

disease.

E. Gut perforation is one of the complications if left untreated.

3. The following are statements regarding food poisoning:

A. *Bacillus cereus* food poisoning of the diarrheal type has a short incubation period.

B. Food contaminated with preformed toxin is the source of clostridial food poisoning.

C. Staphylococcal food poisoning presents primarily with fever.

D. It can be diagnosed by isolating the causative organisms in suspected food items.

E. Broad-spectrum antibiotics are given to shorten the duration of illness.

4. Shigellosis

A. is spread via fecal-oral route.

B. is commonly associated with bacteremia.

C. occurs only after ingestion of food containing large infective dose ($>10^{10}$ organisms).

D. presents with microabscesses in intestinal wall resulting in bleeding.

E. responds to ciprofloxacin therapy.

5. **The following are statements regarding viral hepatitis and their causative viruses:**

    A.   Outbreaks of hepatitis A have been associated with consumption of sewage contaminated oysters.

    B.   Presence of AntiHBc IgM indicates immunity to hepatitis B.

    C.   Hepatitis C virus can be detected in large numbers in stools.

    D.   Hepatitis D is caused by a defective virus which requires HBsAg for transmission.

    E.   Hepatitis E causes fulminant disease in pregnancy.

6. **The following are statements regarding serological markers of hepatitis B:**

    A.   HBcAg is often detected in the blood.

    B.   Presence of anti-HBs in the absence anti-HBc IgG indicates a vaccine type response.

    C.   Anti-HBc IgM rises early in infection and indicates recent infection.

    D.   Presence of anti-HBe indicates high infectivity in hepatitis B carrier.

    E.   Anti-HBc IgG is undetectable in patients who have cleared from the infection.

7. **Hepatitis A**

    A.   is caused by a double-stranded DNA virus.

B.   is often associated with hepatocellular carcinoma.

C.   can be acquired by ingestion of contaminated seafood.

D.   is confirmed by detecting IgM-specific anti-HAV in the blood.

E.   can be prevented by active immunization.

8.   Acute cholangitis

A.   is commonly caused by *Staphylococcus aureus*.

B.   is rarely associated with jaundice.

C.   presents with right hyponchondrial pain

D.   commonly occurs in patients with cholelithiasis.

E.   is associated with bacteremia and septic shock.

9.   Liver abscess

A.   is usually secondary to biliary tract disease.

B.   presents with severe jaundice in almost all cases.

C.   is more frequently found in the left lobe.

D.   can be caused by *Escherichia coli* and *Bacteroides fragilis*.

E.   is treated empirically with 3rd generation cephalosporins and metronidazole.

10.   Rotavirus and Norwalk virus are distinctly different viruses but they share the following characteristics:

A. They are both RNA viruses.

B. Their primary mode of transmission is fecal-oral.

C. They both cause gastroenteritis only in infants.

D. They are easily cultivable in tissue cultures.

E. Large quantities of both viruses are shed in the feces.

6.2.b Questions with answers

1.   The following are statements regarding cholera:

F   A.   It is only caused by *Vibrio cholerae* serotype O1.

F   B.   The causative organism usually invades into the bloodstream.

T   C.   It is due to the heat-labile enterotoxin released by the causative organism.

T   D.   Profuse watery diarrhea and abdominal cramps are the common clinical manifestations.

T   E.   Treatment consists of fluid and electrolyte replacement and doxycycline.

2.   The following are statements regarding typhoid fever:

F   A.   It is caused by *Salmonella paratyphi* A, B and C.

T   B.   Its causative organism multiplies in intestinal lymphoid tissue and excreted in stools.

T   C.   Fever and hepatosplenomegaly are the common clinical manifestations.

F   D.   Stool culture is usually positive in first week of the disease.

T   E.   Gut perforation is one of the complications if left untreated.

3. The following are statements regarding food poisoning:

F   A.   *Bacillus cereus* food poisoning of the diarrheal type has a short incubation period.

F   B.   Food contaminated with preformed toxin is the source of clostridial food poisoning.

F   C.   Staphylococcal food poisoning presents primarily with fever.

T   D.   It can be diagnosed by isolating the causative organisms in suspected food items.

F   E.   Broad-spectrum antibiotics are given to shorten the duration of illness.

4. Shigellosis

T   A.   is spread via fecal-oral route.

F   B.   is commonly associated with bacteremia.

F   C.   occurs only after ingestion of food containing large infective dose ($>10^{10}$ organisms).

T   D.   presents with microabscesses in intestinal wall resulting in bleeding.

T   E.   responds to ciprofloxacin therapy.

5. The following are statements regarding viral hepatitis and their causative viruses:

T   A.   Outbreaks of hepatitis A have been associated with consumption of sewage contaminated oysters.

F   B.   Presence of AntiHBc IgM indicates immunity to hepatitis B.

F   C.   Hepatitis C virus can be detected in large numbers in stools.

T   D.   Hepatitis D is caused by a defective virus which requires HBsAg for transmission.

T   E.   Hepatitis E causes fulminant disease in pregnancy.

6.   The following are statements regarding serological markers of hepatitis B:

F   A.   HBcAg is often detected in the blood.

T   B.   Presence of anti-HBs in the absence anti-HBc IgG indicates a vaccine type response.

T   C.   Anti-HBc IgM rises early in infection and indicates recent infection.

F   D.   Presence of anti-HBe indicates high infectivity in hepatitis B carrier.

F   E.   Anti-HBc IgG is undetectable in patients who have cleared from the infection.

7.   Hepatitis A

F   A.   is caused by a double-stranded DNA virus.

F   B.   is often associated with hepatocellular carcinoma.

T   C.   can be acquired by ingestion of contaminated seafood.

T   D.   is confirmed by detecting IgM-specific anti-HAV in the blood.

T   E.   can be prevented by active immunization.

8. Acute cholangitis

F   A.   is commonly caused by *Staphylococcus aureus*.

F   B.   is rarely associated with jaundice.

T   C.   presents with right hyponchondrial pain

T   D.   commonly occurs in patients with cholelithiasis.

T   E.   is associated with bacteremia and septic shock.

9. Liver abscess

T   A.   is usually secondary to biliary tract disease.

F   B.   presents with severe jaundice in almost all cases.

F   C.   is more frequently found in the left lobe.

T   D.   can be caused by *Escherichia coli* and *Bacteroides fragilis*.

T   E.   is treated empirically with 3rd generation cephalosporins and metronidazole.

10. Rotavirus and Norwalk virus are distinctly different viruses but they share the following characteristics:

T   A.   They are both RNA viruses.

T   B.   Their primary mode of transmission is fecal-oral.

F   C.   They both cause gastroenteritis only in infants.

F   D.   They are easily cultivable in tissue cultures.

T   E.   Large quantities of both viruses are shed in the feces.

7 URINARY SYSTM

7.1 Pathology of Urinary System

7.1.a Questions without answers

1. Causes of respiratory alkalosis include:

A. Excessive mechanical ventilation.

B. Anxiety

C. Subarachniod haemorrage

D. High altitude

E. Pregnancy

2. Regarding respiratory acidosis:

A. Hyperventilation

B. Decreased blood carbon dioxide concentration

C. Increased pH.

D. Myasthenia gravis is a cause of chronic respiratory acidosis

E. Asthma is a cause of chronic respiratory acidosis

3. Metabolic acidosis is associated with

A. aspirin overdose

B. hypokalemia

C. gastric fluid aspiration

D. normal anion gap in diabetic ketoacidosis

E. decreased plasma HCO_3^- level

4. Metabolic alkalosis is associated with

A. effective compensatory mechanism

B. increased respiratory rate

C. severe diarrhea

D. hyperkalemia

E. bicarbonate administration

5. Causes of hypernatremia include:

A. Diabetes insipidus

B. Intake of a hypertonic fluid

C. Ingestion seawater

D. Mineralcorticoid excess

E.   Diabetes mellitus

6.   **Causes of Hyperkalemia include:**

A.   Renal insufficiency

B.   Diuretics

C.   NSAID medications

D.   Addison's disease

E.   Fever

7.   **Common risk factors for urinary tract infection in women:**

A.   Urinary tract obstruction

B.   Pregnancy

C.   Neurogenic bladder

D.   Sexual intercourse

E.   Androgen deficiency

8.   **The following macroscopic and microscopic changes may develop in chronic pyelonephritis:**

A.   Interstitial fibrosis

B.   The minute abscesses

C.   Deformed and dilated calyces

D.   Atrophic and dilated tubules

E. Thyroidisation of the kidney

9. **Causes of acute tubular necrosis include:**

  A. Hypovolemic shock

  B. Septic shock

  C. postpartum hemorrhage

  D. Acute urethritis

  E. Heavy metals

10. **Signs and symptoms of renal failure include:**

  A. Vomiting and/or diarrhea, which may lead to dehydration

  B. Weight loss

  C. Dyspnoea

  D. Leg edema

  E. Hyporkalemia

11. **Biochemical changes in acute renal failure include:**

  A. Hyperkalemia

  B. Hypocalcemia

  C. Hyperuricemia

  D. Alkalosis

  E. Hyponatremia

12. **Causes of chronic renal failure include:**

A. Hypertension

B. Severe burns

C. Chronic pyelonephritis

D. Hyperuricemia

E. Acute glomerulonephritis

13. **The following conditions predispose to urolithiasis:**

A. High dietary intake of animal sodium

B. Cola drinks

C. Gout

D. Avitaminosis A

E. Dehydration

14. **Signs and symptoms of renal stones include:**

A. Excruciating intermittent pain that radiates from the flank to the groin or to the genital area and inner thigh

B. Urinary urgency

C. Hematuria

D. Hypertension

E. Nausea and vomiting

15. **Hematuria is a characteristic clinical feature of all of the following diseases:**

    A. Urinary schistosomiasis

    B. Lipoid nephritis

    C. Papillary necrosis

    D. Renal cell carcinoma

    E. Bladder carcinoma

16. **The following are statements regarding glomerular diseases**

    A. It is one of the most common causes of chronic renal failure

    B. It is induced by antigen-antibody reactions.

    C. Antigen-antibody deposition in the glomerulus is a major pathway of glomerular injury.

    D. The loss of glomerular barrier function is manifested by proteinuria.

    E. Epithelial cell injury of glomeruli can be induced by antibodies to visceral epithelial cell antigens.

17. **The following are statements regarding nephrotic syndrome:**

    A. It refers to a clinical complex that includes massive protienuria.

    B. Among children it may often be associated with a systemic disease.

    C. The most frequent systemic cause of the nephrotic syndrome is hypertension

D. The most important of the primary glomerular lesions that lead to nephrotic syndrome are membranous GN, and lipoid nephrosis.

E. Generalized edema, is the most obvious clinical manifestation.

18. **Signs and Symptoms of Renal cell carcinoma include:**

A. Gross or microscopic hematuria

B. A palpable mass

C. Hypertension

D. Hypocalcemia

E. Paraneoplastic syndromes

19. **The following are statements regarding morphology of renal cell carcinoma:**

A. It is usually solitary

B. The cut surface of clear cell renal cell carcinomas is yellow to orange to gray-white colour.

C. The margins of the tumor are well defined

D. The tumor may invades the renal vein

E. Direct invasion to adrenal gland.

20. **Signs and Symptoms of bladder carcinoma include**

A. Unexplained hematuria (gross or microscopic).

B. Urinary obstruction

C. Anemia

D. Dysuria, burning and frequency

E. Pelvic pain

7.1.b Questions with answers

1.   Causes of respiratory alkalosis include:

T   A.   Excessive mechanical ventilation.

T   B.   Anxiety

T   C.   Subarachniod haemorrage

T   D.   High altitude

T   E.   Pregnancy

2.   Regarding respiratory acidosis:

F   A.   Hyperventilation

F   B.   Decreased blood carbon dioxide concentration

F   C.   Increased pH.

F   D.   Myasthenia gravis is a cause of chronic respiratory acidosis

T   E.   Asthma is a cause of chronic respiratory acidosis

3.   Metabolic acidosis is associated with

T   A.   aspirin overdose

F   B.   hypokalemia

F   C.   gastric fluid aspiration

F D. normal anion gap in diabetic ketoacidosis

T E. decreased plasma HCO_3^- level

4. Metabolic alkalosis is associated with

F A. effective compensatory mechanism

F B. increased respiratory rate

F C. severe diarrhea

F D. hyperkalemia

T E. bicarbonate administration

5. Causes of hypernatremia include:

T A. Diabetes insipidus

T B. Intake of a hypertonic fluid

T C. Ingestion seawater

T D. Mineralcorticoid excess

F E. Diabetes mellitus

6. Causes of Hyperkalemia include:

T A. Renal insufficiency

T B. Diuretics

T C. NSAID medications

T D. Addison's disease

F   E.   Fever

7.   Common risk factors for urinary tract infection in women:

T   A.   Urinary tract obstruction

T   B.   Pregnancy

T   C.   Neurogenic bladder

T   D.   Sexual intercourse

F   E.   Androgen deficiency

8.   The following macroscopic and microscopic changes may develop in chronic pyelonephritis:

T   A.   Interstitial fibrosis

F   B.   The minute abscesses

T   C.   Deformed and dilated calyces

T   D.   Atrophic and dilated tubules

T   E.   Thyroidisation of the kidney

9.   Causes of acute tubular necrosis include:

T   A.   Hypovolemic shock

T   B.   Septic shock

T   C.   postpartum hemorrhage

F   D.   Acute urethritis

T   E.   Heavy metals

10.   **Signs and symptoms of renal failure include:**

T   A.   Vomiting and/or diarrhea, which may lead to dehydration

T   B.   Weight loss

T   C.   Dyspnoea

T   D.   Leg edema

F   E.   Hyporkalemia

11.   **Biochemical changes in acute renal failure include:**

T   A.   Hyperkalemia

F   B.   Hypocalcemia

T   C.   Hyperuricemia

F   D.   Alkalosis

T   E.   Hyponatremia

12.   **Causes of chronic renal failure include:**

T   A.   Hypertension

F   B.   Severe burns

T   C.   Chronic pyelonephritis

T   D.   Hyperuricemia

F   E.   Acute glomerulonephritis

13. **The following conditions predispose to urolithiasis:**

T A. High dietary intake of animal sodium

T B. Cola drinks

T C. Gout

T D. Avitaminosis A

T E. Dehydration

14. **Signs and symptoms of renal stones include:**

T A. Excruciating intermittent pain that radiates from the flank to the groin or to the genital area and inner thigh

T B. Urinary urgency

T C. Hematuria

F D. Hypertension

T E. Nausea and vomiting

15. **Hematuria is a characteristic clinical feature of all of the following diseases:**

T A. Urinary schistosomiasis

F B. Lipoid nephritis

T C. Papillary necrosis

T D. Renal cell carcinoma

T E. Bladder carcinoma

16. The following are statements regarding glomerular diseases

T A. It is one of the most common causes of chronic renal failure

T B. It is induced by antigen-antibody reactions.

T C. Antigen-antibody deposition in the glomerulus is a major pathway of glomerular injury.

T D. The loss of glomerular barrier function is manifested by proteinuria.

T E. Epithelial cell injury of glomeruli can be induced by antibodies to visceral epithelial cell antigens.

17. The following are statements regarding nephrotic syndrome:

T A. It refers to a clinical complex that includes massive protienuria.

F B. Among children it may often be associated with a systemic disease.

F C. The most frequent systemic cause of the nephrotic syndrome is hypertension

T D. The most important of the primary glomerular lesions that lead to nephrotic syndrome are membranous GN, and lipoid nephrosis.

T E. Generalized edema, is the most obvious clinical manifestation.

18. Signs and Symptoms of Renal cell carcinoma include:

T A. Gross or microscopic hematuria

T B. A palpable mass

T   C.   Hypertension

F   D.   Hypocalcemia

T   E.   Paraneoplastic syndromes

19.   The following are statements regarding morphology of renal cell carcinoma:

T   A.   It is usually solitary

T   B.   The cut surface of clear cell renal cell carcinomas is yellow to orange to gray-white colour.

T   C.   The margins of the tumor are well defined

T   D.   The tumor may invades the renal vein

T   E.   Direct invasion to adrenal gland.

20.   Signs and Symptoms of bladder carcinoma include

T   A.   Unexplained hematuria (gross or microscopic).

T   B.   Urinary obstruction

T   C.   Anemia

T   D.   Dysuria, burning and frequency

T   E.   Pelvic pain

7.2 Microbiology of Urinary System

7.2.a Questions without answers

1.   Acute bacterial prostatitis

A.   is commonly caused by *Staphylococcus aureus*.

B.   presents with a sudden onset of fever and acute urinary retention.

C.   is only confirmed by culturing expressed prostatic secretion.

D.   is treated with intravenous broad-spectrum beta-lactams in severe cases.

E.   develops into abscess as a complication.

2.   Urethritis

A.   may occur following catheterization.

B.   of the non-gonococcal type is caused by *Chlamydia trachomatis*.

C.   presents with dysuria and purulent urethral discharge.

D.   is diagnosed by culturing urethral discharge on CLED agar.

E.   due to gonococcus is treated with doxycycline.

3. **The following are statements regarding urinary tract infection:**

    A. It is characterized by presence of pyuria and significant bacteruria.

    B. The causative organisms gain entry into urinary system mainly via bloodstream.

    C. *Staphylococcus saprophyticus* is a common causative organism in young sexually active women.

    D. Dysuria and frequency of micturition are among the clinical manifestations.

    E. Quinolones are one of the antibiotics used in the treatment.

4. **The following are statements regarding hospital-acquired urinary tract infection:**

    A. Catheterization is a common predisposing factor.

    B. *Pseudomonas aeruginosa* is one of the common causative organisms.

    C. Urine for culture should be taken from the urine bag.

    D. It is a common source of Gram-positive bacteremia in hospitalized patients.

    E. It results in prolonged hospital stay.

5. **The following are statements regarding laboratory diagnosis of urinary tract infection:**

    A. Urine samples should be collected immediately after

starting antibiotic therapy.

B.   Significant bacteriuria is defined as the presence of >
     10^5 colony forming units/mm^3 urine.

C.   Positive results obtained from an overnight urine culture
     should be interpreted with caution.

D.   The presence of 10^2 cfu /ml in a sample obtained from
     urine bag is significant.

E.   Mixed growth of organisms in mid-stream urine culture
     usually indicates severe infection.

7.2.b Questions with answers

1.   Acute bacterial prostatitis

F   A.   is commonly caused by *Staphylococcus aureus*.

T   B.   presents with a sudden onset of fever and acute urinary retention.

F   C.   is only confirmed by culturing expressed prostatic secretion.

T   D.   is treated with intravenous broad-spectrum beta-lactams in severe cases.

T   E.   develops into abscess as a complication.

2.   Urethritis

T   A.   may occur following catheterization.

T   B.   of the non-gonococcal type is caused by *Chlamydia trachomatis*.

T   C.   presents with dysuria and purulent urethral discharge.

F   D.   is diagnosed by culturing urethral discharge on CLED agar.

F   E.   due to gonococcus is treated with doxycycline.

3.   The following are statements regarding urinary tract infection:

F   A.   It is characterized by presence of pyuria and significant bacteruria.

F   B.   The causative organisms gain entry into urinary system mainly via bloodstream.

T   C.   *Staphylococcus saprophyticus* is a common causative organism in young sexually active women.

T   D.   Dysuria and frequency of micturition are among the clinical manifestations.

T   E.   Quinolones are one of the antibiotics used in the treatment.

4.   The following are statements regarding hospital-acquired urinary tract infection:

T   A.   Catheterization is a common predisposing factor.

T   B.   *Pseudomonas aeruginosa* is one of the common causative organisms.

F   C.   Urine for culture should be taken from the urine bag.

F   D.   It is a common source of Gram-positive bacteremia in hospitalized patients.

T   E.   It results in prolonged hospital stay.

5.   The following are statements regarding laboratory diagnosis of urinary tract infection:

F   A.   Urine samples should be collected immediately after starting antibiotic therapy.

T   B.   Significant bacteriuria is defined as the presence of >

10^5 colony forming units/mm^3 urine.

T C.   Positive results obtained from an overnight urine culture should be interpreted with caution.

F D.   The presence of 10^2 cfu /ml in a sample obtained from urine bag is significant.

F E.   Mixed growth of organisms in mid-stream urine culture usually indicates severe infection.

8 REPRODUCTIVE SYSTEM

8.1 Pathology of Reproductive System

8.1.a Questions without answers

1. The following are statements regarding lichen simplex chronicus

    A.   It marked by epithelial thickening with significant surface hyperkeratosis

    B.   Leukoplakia is characteristic.

    C.   Epithelium may show increased mitotic activity

    D.   The hyperplastic epithelial changed show atypia

    E.   Increased predisposition to cancer is generally associated

2. The following are statements regarding neoplasms of the vulva

    A.   Majority of cases are adenocarcimoma type.

    B.   Perinuclear cytoplasmic vacuolation is charactristic morphology.

    C.   There is strong association with at least two types of HPV.

D.   HPV-positive neoplasms tend to be poorly differentiated

E.   Smoking is a risk factor

3.   **Predisposing factors of cervical carcinoma include:**

A.   Early age at 1st intercourse

B.   Multiple sexual partners

C.   Smoking

D.   Chlamydia infection

E.   Nulliparity

4.   **The following are statements regarding precancerous changes of cervical carcinoma:**

A.   Cervical Intraepithelial Neoplasia (CIN) I resembles mild dysplasia

B.   Cervical Intraepithelial Neoplasia (CIN) II resembles severe dysplasia

C.   Cervical Intraepithelial Neoplasia (CIN) III resembles carcinoma in situ

D.   CIN I is characterized by koilocytotic changes mostly in the superficial layers of the epithelium.

E.   CIN II affects most layers of the epithelium.

5.   **The following are statements regarding symptoms and signs of cervical carcinoma**

A. CIN lesions are usually symptomatic

B. Early cervical cancer usually manifests as irregular vaginal bleeding

C. Bleeding is most often postcoital

D. Leukorrhea

E. Back pain is present in widespread cancer

6. **The following are statements regarding leiomyoma (Fibroid of uterus)**

A. They are benign tumors arise from the smooth muscle cells in the myometrium

B. Genetic influence is a cause

C. Oral contraceptives are risk factor

D. Bundles of smooth muscle cells duplicating the normal myometrium are morphological findings

E. Most frequent manifestation is menorrhagia with or without metrorrhagia

7. **Risk factors of Endometrial carcinoma include:**

A. Hypertension

B. Polycystic ovary syndrome

C. Multiple pregnancies

D. Breast cancer

E. Lack of exercise

8. **The following are statements regarding endometrial carcinoma:**

    A. It is usually squamous cell carcinoma.

    B. Infertility is a risk factor.

    C. It appears mostly between the ages of 55 and 65 years.

    D. In stage III, the tumor is beyond the uterus but within the true pelvis.

    E. The uterus can be palpable in advanced cases.

9. **The following are statements regarding ovarian cancer:**

    A. In few cases, the symptoms persist for several months before being recognized and diagnosed

    B. Bloating, abdominal or pelvic pain are most typical symptoms

    C. Multiple pregnancies is a risk factor

    D. Ovarian cancer at its early stages is difficult to diagnose until it spreads

    E. Fluid from the abdominal cavity is useful in diagnosis

10. **The following are statements regarding morphological differences of the serous ovarian tumour**

    A. They are commonly malignant

    B. There is bilateral involvement of ovary

    C. Majority are uniloculated

D. The borderline tumors are more complex papillary structure

E. The malignant tumors are large solid areas with areas of haemorrhage and necrosis

11. **The following are statements regarding morphology of mucinous cystadenocarcinoma**

A. Cysts and glands lined by atypical epithelium of intestinal type.

B. Benign borderline, and malignant components

C. The borderline appeared as thin and branching papillae

D. Numerous foci of infiltrating anaplastic tumor cells

E. Extensive necrosis with "amputated" glands

12. **The following are statements regarding teratoma**

A. It contains organs and one or more tissues normally found in organs.

B. They are the result of abnormal development of pluripotent cells

C. Mature teratomas generally are malignant

D. ultrasound imaging helps in diagnosis

E. The most commonly diagnosed fetal teratomas are sacrococcygeal teratoma

13. **The following are statements regarding morphology of seminomas**

A. Testicular atrophy is characteristic.

B. The usual presentation is a lobulated, single to multinodular mass, confined to the testis but with a tendency to bulge into the surrounding parenchyma

C. Seminomas often have a diffuse, sheetlike pattern

D. Ccribriform is common histologic variants of seminomas

E. Dense fibrous septae are rare

14. **The following are statements regarding testicular cancer**

A. Majority of cases are seen before the age of 15 years

B. It can be derived from any cell type found in the testicles

C. A lump or swelling in the testes is one of first signs

D. Gynecomastia is a symptom

E. It has poor prognosis

15. **The following are statements regarding prostate Cancer**

A. It is the most common male cancer.

B. Nodular, firm, and enlarged prostate on digital rectal examination.

C. Elevated Prostate specific antigen (PSA) but decreased alkaline phosphatase

D. Usually the lateral lobes of the prostate are affected

E. Frequency of urination, hesitancy, dribbling, and frequent nighttime urination are the major urinary symptoms

16. **The following are statements regarding benign prostatic hyperplasia**

    A. It is the most common cause of male urinary tract obstruction.

    B. Increased levels of testosterone is the cause

    C. Enlarged prostate on digital rectal examination.

    D. Decreased prostate specific antigen (PSA).

    E. Usually the central portion of the prostate is affected

17. **Symptoms of orchitis include:**

    A. Ejaculation of blood

    B. Hematuria

    C. Severe pain

    D. Visible swelling of a testicle

    E. Inguinal lymph nodes on the affected side

18. **The following are statements regarding fibroadenoma**

    A. The typical case is the presence of a painless, firm, solitary, mobile, slowly growing lump.

    B. It arises in the terminal duct lobular unit of the breast

    C. It appears after the age of thirty years

    D. Needle biopsy is diagnostic

    E. Morphology consists of abundant stromal cells, which appear as bare bipolar nuclei

19. **Risk factors of breast cancer include:**

    A. Obesity

    B. Longer reproductive span

    C. Multiple pregnancies

    D. Later age at first pregnancy

    E. BRCA1 and BRCA2 genes

20. **The following are statements regarding invasive ductal carcinoma" IDC" of breast:**

    A. It is the commonest form of breast cancer

    B. The lump is hard, irregular and palpable

    C. Axillary mass is uncommon

    D. Scirrhous carcinoma is the commonest type

    E. Histology shows infiltrating clusters of malignant cells in a dense, fibrous stroma

8.1.b Questions with answers

1.   The following are statements regarding lichen simplex chronicus

T   A.   It marked by epithelial thickening with significant surface hyperkeratosis

T   B.   Leukoplakia is characteristic.

T   C.   Epithelium may show increased mitotic activity

F   D.   The hyperplastic epithelial changed show atypia

F   E.   Increased predisposition to cancer is generally associated

2.   The following are statements regarding neoplasms of the vulva

F   A.   Majority of cases are adenocarcimoma type.

T   B.   Perinuclear cytoplasmic vacuolation is charactristic morphology.

T   C.   There is strong association with at least two types of HPV.

T   D.   HPV-positive neoplasms tend to be poorly differentiated

T   E.   Smoking is a risk factor

3.   Predisposing factors of cervical carcinoma include:

T   A.   Early age at 1st intercourse

T   B.   Multiple sexual partners

T   C.   Smoking

T   D.   Chlamydia infection

F   E.   Nulliparity

4.   The following are statements regarding precancerous changes of cervical carcinoma:

T   A.   Cervical Intraepithelial Neoplasia (CIN) I resembles mild dysplasia

F   B.   Cervical Intraepithelial Neoplasia (CIN) II resembles severe dysplasia

T   C.   Cervical Intraepithelial Neoplasia (CIN) III resembles carcinoma in situ

T   D.   CIN I is characterized by koilocytotic changes mostly in the superficial layers of the epithelium.

T   E.   CIN II affects most layers of the epithelium.

5.   The following are statements regarding symptoms and signs of cervical carcinoma

F   A.   CIN lesions are usually symptomatic

T   B.   Early cervical cancer usually manifests as irregular vaginal bleeding

T   C.   Bleeding is most often postcoital

T   D.   Leukorrhea

T   E.   Back pain is present in widespread cancer

6. **The following are statements regarding leiomyoma (Fibroid of uterus)**

T   A.   They are benign tumors arise from the smooth muscle cells in the myometrium

T   B.   Genetic influence is a cause

T   C.   Oral contraceptives are risk factor

T   D.   Bundles of smooth muscle cells duplicating the normal myometrium are morphological findings

T   E.   Most frequent manifestation is menorrhagia with or without metrorrhagia

7. **Risk factors of Endometrial carcinoma include:**

T   A.   Hypertension

T   B.   Polycystic ovary syndrome

F   C.   Multiple pregnancies

T   D.   Breast cancer

T   E.   Lack of exercise

8. **The following are statements regarding endometrial carcinoma:**

F   A.   It is usually squamous cell carcinoma.

T   B.   Infertility is a risk factor.

T   C.   It appears mostly between the ages of 55 and 65 years.

T   D.   In stage III, the tumor is beyond the uterus but within the true pelvis.

T   E.   The uterus can be palpable in advanced cases.

9.   The following are statements regarding ovarian cancer:

F   A.   In few cases, the symptoms persist for several months before being recognized and diagnosed

T   B.   Bloating, abdominal or pelvic pain are most typical symptoms

F   C.   Multiple pregnancies is a risk factor

T   D.   Ovarian cancer at its early stages is difficult to diagnose until it spreads

T   E.   Fluid from the abdominal cavity is useful in diagnosis

10.   The following are statements regarding morphological differences of the serous ovarian tumour

F   A.   They are commonly malignant

T   B.   There is bilateral involvement of ovary

T   C.   Majority are uniloculated

T   D.   The borderline tumors are more complex papillary structure

T   E.   The malignant tumors are large solid areas with areas of haemorrhage and necrosis

11.   The following are statements regarding morphology of mucinous cystadenocarcinoma

T   A.   Cysts and glands lined by atypical epithelium of intestinal type.

T   B.   Benign borderline, and malignant components

T   C.   The borderline appeared as thin and branching papillae

T   D.   Numerous foci of infiltrating anaplastic tumor cells

T   E.   Extensive necrosis with "amputated" glands

12.   The following are statements regarding teratoma

F   A.   It contains organs and one or more tissues normally found in organs.

T   B.   They are the result of abnormal development of pluripotent cells

F   C.   Mature teratomas generally are malignant

T   D.   ultrasound imaging helps in diagnosis

T   E.   The most commonly diagnosed fetal teratomas are sacrococcygeal teratoma

13.   The following are statements regarding morphology of seminomas

F   A.   Testicular atrophy is characteristic.

T   B.   The usual presentation is a lobulated, single to multinodular mass, confined to the testis but with a tendency to bulge into the surrounding parenchyma

T   C.   Seminomas often have a diffuse, sheetlike pattern

F   D.   Ccribriform is common histologic variants of seminomas

F   E.   Dense fibrous septae are rare

14.   The following are statements regarding testicular cancer

F   A.   Majority of cases are seen before the age of 15 years

T   B.   It can be derived from any cell type found in the testicles

T   C.   A lump or swelling in the testes is one of first signs

T   D.   Gynecomastia is a symptom

F   E.   It has poor prognosis

15.   The following are statements regarding prostate Cancer

T   A.   It is the most common male cancer.

T   B.   Nodular, firm, and enlarged prostate on digital rectal examination.

F   C.   Elevated Prostate specific antigen (PSA) but decreased alkaline phosphatase

T   D.   Usually the lateral lobes of the prostate are affected

T   E.   Frequency of urination, hesitancy, dribbling, and frequent nighttime urination are the major urinary symptoms

16.   The following are statements regarding benign prostatic hyperplasia

T   A.   It is the most common cause of male urinary tract obstruction.

T   B.   Increased levels of testosterone is the cause

T   C.   Enlarged prostate on digital rectal examination.

F   D.   Decreased prostate specific antigen (PSA).

T   E.   Usually the central portion of the prostate is affected

17. **Symptoms of orchitis include:**

T   A.   Ejaculation of blood

T   B.   Hematuria

T   C.   Severe pain

T   D.   Visible swelling of a testicle

T   E.   Inguinal lymph nodes on the affected side

18. **The following are statements regarding fibroadenoma**

T   A.   The typical case is the presence of a painless, firm, solitary, mobile, slowly growing lump.

T   B.   It arises in the terminal duct lobular unit of the breast

F   C.   It appears after the age of thirty years

T   D.   Needle biopsy is diagnostic

T   E.   Morphology consists of abundant stromal cells, which appear as bare bipolar nuclei

19. **Risk factors of breast cancer include:**

T   A.   Obesity

T   B.   Longer reproductive span

F   C.   Multiple pregnancies

T   D.   Later age at first pregnancy

T   E.   BRCA1 and BRCA2 genes

20. The following are statements regarding invasive ductal carcinoma" IDC" of breast:

T   A.   It is the commonest form of breast cancer

T   B.   The lump is hard, irregular and palpable

F   C.   Axillary mass is uncommon

T   D.   Scirrhous carcinoma is the commonest type

T   E.   Histology shows infiltrating clusters of malignant cells in a dense, fibrous stroma

8.2 Microbiology of Reproductive System

8.2.a Questions without answers

1. The following are statements regarding sexually transmitted diseases:

A.   Human papilloma virus types 6 and 11 cause condylomata lata.

B.   *Haemophilus ducreyi* infection presents with painful soft chancre.

C.   Both the primary and secondary syphilis lesions are not infectious.

D.   Presence of intracellular Gram-negative diplococci in the urethral discharge provides a presumptive diagnosis of gonorrhoea.

E.   Penicillin is used in the treatment of *Chlamydia trachomatis* genital infections.

2. Bacterial vaginosis

A.   is due to the overgrowth of lactobacilli.

B.   is characterized by profuse vaginal discharge of pH<4.5.

C.   is associated with preterm low birth weight delivery.

D.   is diagnosed based on the presence of clue cells in high vaginal swabs.

E.   is treated with metronidazole.

3.   **The following are statements regarding serological tests for syphilis:**

A.   VDRL false positive can be seen patients with collagen vascular disease.

B.   FTA-Abs test remains positive in late syphilis.

C.   TPHA test is used as an indicator of therapeutic response.

D.   All serological tests become negative after penicillin therapy.

E.   Presence of FTA-Abs IgG in neonates confirms the diagnosis of congenital syphilis.

4.   **Gonorrhoea**

A.   is a sexually-transmitted disease.

B.   is caused by fastidious extracellular Gram-positive diplococci.

C.   in men, usually presents with purulent urethral discharge associated with dysuria.

D.   is rarely associated co-infection with *Chlamydia trachomatis.*

E.   is treated with doxycycline.

5.   **The following are statements regarding genital herpes:**

  A.   It is usually caused by herpes simplex type 2.

  B.   Primary genital lesions are seen approximately one week after the infection.

  C.   It presents with painful vesiculo-ulcerative lesions of the penis and cervix.

  D.   Recurrent genital herpes is usually more severe and of longer duration.

  E.   It causes laryngeal papilloma in babies born to infected mothers.

6.   **The following are statements regarding human papillomavirus infection:**

  A.   Infections with types 16 and 18 are associated with cervical cancer.

  B.   Genital warts usually regress spontaneously.

  C.   The virus alone without the co-factor is responsible for its progression to cancer.

  D.   It is characterized by the presence of 'koilocytes'

  E.   HPV vaccines available are effective against established infections.

7.   **A 25-year-old nurse has needle-stick injury with blood of a known HIV-positive drug addict. Six months later, EIA test was positive, a repeat EIA was equivocal but Western blot was negative. The nurse**

A.   probably requires immediate antiretroviral therapy.

B.   is in the window between acute infection with HIV and seroconversion.

C.   is probably not infected with HIV.

D.   may be infected with drug-resistant strain of HIV2.

E.   may be a long term non-progressor.

8.   **The following are statements regarding pathogenesis of HIV infection:**

A.   Th cells are directly killed by the HIV.

B.   CD4+ bearing cells are induced to undergo apoptosis.

C.   T cell replenishment is unimpaired as the stem cells are not infected.

D.   Antigen processing and presentation are not affected.

E.   HIV produces gp120 immunosuppressive virus-coded molecules.

9.   **Congenital rubella syndrome**

A.   is a complication of maternal infection occurring in 3rd trimester of pregnancy.

B.   is characterized by classical triad of cataract, deafness and patent ductus arteriosus.

C.   is confirmed by detecting specific IgG in cord blood.

D.   is associated with insulin-dependent diabetes mellitus later in life.

E.   is prevented by vaccinating mothers during the 1st trimester of pregnancy.

10.   **The following are statements regarding puerperal sepsis:**

A.   The causative organisms usually originate from the mother's own fecal flora.

B.   *Streptococcus* group B is one of the causative organisms.

C.   Presence of retained placenta fragments is one of the predisposing factors.

D.   Fever and offensive vaginal discharge are among the clinical presentations.

E.   Antibiotic therapy is usually not necessary.

8.2.b Questions with answers

1. The following are statements regarding sexually transmitted diseases:

F A.   Human papilloma virus types 6 and 11 cause
        condylomata lata.

T B.   *Haemophilus ducreyi* infection presents with painful soft
        chancre.

F C.   Both the primary and secondary syphilis lesions are not
        infectious.

T D.   Presence of intracellular Gram-negative diplococci in
        the urethral discharge provides a presumptive diagnosis
        of gonorrhoea.

F E.   Penicillin is used in the treatment of *Chlamydia trachomatis*
        genital infections.

2. Bacterial vaginosis

F A.   is due to the overgrowth of lactobacilli.

F B.   is characterized by profuse vaginal discharge of pH<4.5.

T C.   is associated with preterm low birth weight delivery.

T D.   is diagnosed based on the presence of clue cells in high
        vaginal swabs.

T   E.   is treated with metronidazole.

3. The following are statements regarding serological tests for syphilis:

T   A.   VDRL false positive can be seen patients with collagen vascular disease.

T   B.   FTA-Abs test remains positive in late syphilis.

F   C.   TPHA test is used as an indicator of therapeutic response.

F   D.   All serological tests become negative after penicillin therapy.

F   E.   Presence of FTA-Abs IgG in neonates confirms the diagnosis of congenital syphilis.

4. Gonorrhoea

T   A.   is a sexually-transmitted disease.

F   B.   is caused by fastidious extracellular Gram-positive diplococci.

T   C.   in men, usually presents with purulent urethral discharge associated with dysuria.

F   D.   is rarely associated co-infection with *Chlamydia trachomatis.*

F   E.   is treated with doxycycline.

5. The following are statements regarding genital herpes:

T   A.   It is usually caused by herpes simplex type 2.

T   B.   Primary genital lesions are seen approximately one week after the infection.

T   C.   It presents with painful vesiculo-ulcerative lesions of the penis and cervix.

F   D.   Recurrent genital herpes is usually more severe and of longer duration.

F   E.   It causes laryngeal papilloma in babies born to infected mothers.

6. The following are statements regarding human papillomavirus infection:

T   A.   Infections with types 16 and 18 are associated with cervical cancer.

F   B.   Genital warts usually regress spontaneously.

F   C.   The virus alone without the co-factor is responsible for its progression to cancer.

T   D.   It is characterized by the presence of 'koilocytes'

F   E.   HPV vaccines available are effective against established infections.

7. A 25-year-old nurse has needle-stick injury with blood of a known HIV-positive drug addict. Six months later, EIA test was positive, a repeat EIA was equivocal but Western blot was negative. The nurse

F   A.   probably requires immediate antiretroviral therapy.

F B. is in the window between acute infection with HIV and seroconversion.

T C. is probably not infected with HIV.

F D. may be infected with drug-resistant strain of HIV2.

F E. may be a long term non-progressor.

8. **The following are statements regarding pathogenesis of HIV infection:**

T A. Th cells are directly killed by the HIV.

T B. CD4+ bearing cells are induced to undergo apoptosis.

F C. T cell replenishment is unimpaired as the stem cells are not infected.

F D. Antigen processing and presentation are not affected.

T E. HIV produces gp120 immunosuppressive virus-coded molecules.

9. **Congenital rubella syndrome**

F A. is a complication of maternal infection occurring in 3rd trimester of pregnancy.

T B. is characterized by classical triad of cataract, deafness and patent ductus arteriosus.

F C. is confirmed by detecting specific IgG in cord blood.

T D. is associated with insulin-dependent diabetes mellitus later in life.

F E. is prevented by vaccinating mothers during the 1st

trimester of pregnancy.

10.   The following are statements regarding puerperal sepsis:

T   A.   The causative organisms usually originate from the mother's own fecal flora.

T   B.   *Streptococcus* group B is one of the causative organisms.

T   C.   Presence of retained placenta fragments is one of the predisposing factors.

T   D.   Fever and offensive vaginal discharge are among the clinical presentations.

F   E.   Antibiotic therapy is usually not necessary.

9 ENDOCRINE SYSTEM

9.1 Pathology of Endocrine System

9.1.a Questions without answers

1. **The following are statements regarding thyroid diseases:**

   A. Thyroid carcinoma is more frequent in females than males.

   B. Lymphatic metastasis frequently occur in follicular thyroid carcinoma.

   C. Medullary thyroid carcinoma produces calcitonin.

   D. Atrial fiibrillation is a complication of thyrotoxicosis.

   E. Secondary hypercholesterolemia is a feature of hypothyroidism.

2. **The following are statements regarding thyroid diseases:**

   A. Graves disease is more common in females.

B. Hashimoto's thyroiditis is the most common cause of cretinism.

C. In Graves disease, the thyroid gland is markedly enlarged and irregular.

D. The most frequent cause of diffuse goitre is iodine deficiency.

E. Compression on the trachea is a complication of multinodular goiter.

3. **The following are statements regarding Graves disease**

A. Blood levels of thyroid stimulating hormone (TSH) is elevated

B. Heart failure is a complication

C. Proptosis is one of its feature

D. Basal metabolic rate is increased

E. It frequently presents as a solitary thyroid nodule

4. **The following are statements regarding thyroid cancer**

A. It is rarely found in a euthyroid patient.

B. Papillary thyroid cancer often found in young females

C. Majority of cases are follicular thyroid cancer

D. Anaplastic thyroid cancer is responsive well to treatment

E. Fine needle aspiration is diagnostic

5. **The following are statements regarding papillary thyroid carcinoma**

A.   It is the most common type of thyroid cancer

B.   it is more likely to invade blood vessels

C.   Orphan Annie eye nuclear inclusions are characteristic histological finding

D.   Chest x rays are commonly performed in diagnosis

E.   Thyroglobulin is used as a tumor marker for well-differentiated papillary thyroid cancer

6.   **The following are statements regarding acromegaly**

A.   It is a syndrome that results when the anterior pituitary gland produces excess growth hormone before epiphyseal plate closure at puberty

B.   It is easy to diagnose in the early stages

C.   It is often associated with gigantism

D.   Hypertension is a complication

E.   Insulin-like growth factor 1 (IGF-1) provides the most sensitive lab test for the diagnosis of acromegaly

7.   **Signs and symptoms of Cushing's syndrome include:**

A.   Weight loss

B.   irritability

C.   Muscle and bone weakness

D.   Diabetes mellitus

E.   Hypotension

8. **Causes of syndrome of inappropriate antidiuretic hormone secretion include:**

    A. Meningitis

    B. Subarachnoid hemorrhage

    C. Lung cancer

    D. Brain abscess

    E. Guillain-Barré syndrome

9. **The following are statements regarding hypercalcaemia**

    A. If caused by primary hyperparathyroidism, serum phosphate is low.

    B. Chronic renal failure is a common cause.

    C. There is polyuria.

    D. Renal stone formation is a complication.

    E. Medullary carcinoma of the thyroid is a cause.

10. **The following are statements regarding adrenal diseases:**

    A. Auto-immune disease is a cause of adrenal hypofunction.

    B. Hyperpigmentation occurs in primary adrenal failure.

    C. Adrenal insufficiency causes hyponatremia.

    D. Hypertension is a feature of Conn's syndrome.

    E. Pheochromocytoma causes hypotension.

11. **The following are statements regarding pheochromocytoma**

    A. It is a tumor of chromaffin cells that arises inside the adrenal glands

    B. Hypotention is a feature

    C. Men are likely to inherit the disease more than women

    D. This syndrome is mostly occur in between the ages of 30 to 60.

    E. Excess sweating is a presentation

12. **The following are statements regarding hyperaldosteronism**

    A. Most cases of primary hyperaldosteronism are caused by a cancerous tumor of the adrenal gland.

    B. The disease is common above age of 60

    C. Cirrhosis of the liver is a cause of secondary hyperaldosteronism

    D. Heart failure is a cause of secondary hyperaldosteronism

    E. High serum potassium is a symptom

13. **Characteristic symptoms of Addison's crisis include:**

    A. Sudden penetrating pain in the legs, lower back or abdomen

    B. Severe vomiting but without diarrhea

    C. Hyperglycemia

    D. Hypernatremia

    E. Hypocalcemia

14. **Causes of Conn syndrome include:**

A.   Adrenal carcinoma

B.   Adrenal hypoplasia

C.   Adrenal adenoma

D.   Dexamethasone-suppressible hyperaldosteronism

E.   Disorders of the renin-angiotensin system

15. **Features of Cushing's syndrome include:**

A.   Hypokalemia.

B.   Metabolic acidosis.

C.   Postural hypotension.

D.   Truncal obesity.

E.   Hirsutism.

16. **The following are statements regarding diabetes mellitus (DM)**

A.   Type 2 diabetes mellitus is characterized by loss of the insulin-producing beta cells of the islets of Langerhans in the pancreas

B.   Type 1 diabetes is of the immune-mediated nature

C.   Type 1 diabetes mellitus is characterized by insulin resistance

D.   Gestational diabetes mellitus resembles type 2 diabetes in several respects

E.   Prediabetes indicates a condition that occurs when a person's blood glucose levels are higher than normal but not high enough for a diagnosis of type 2 DM

17. **The following are statements regarding diabetes mellitus:**

A. Type 2 diabetes is more common in children.

B. Diagnosis is by measurement of HBA_{1c} level.

C. Hyperthyroidism is a cause.

D. Deposition of amyloid in the islet of Langerhans is seen in type 2 diabetes.

E. Obesity is a predisposing factor for type 2 diabetes.

18. **The following are statements regarding acute complications of diabetes mellitus**

A. Elevated levels of ketone bodies in the blood decrease the blood's pH leading to diabetic ketoacidosis

B. Severe abdominal pain is common in diabetic ketoacidosis.

C. Hyperosmolar nonketotic state is sharing many symptoms with diabetic ketoacidosis

D. Electrolyte imbalances are common in hyperosmolar nonketotic

E. The patient may become agitated, sweaty, weak in hypoglycemia

19. **The following are statements regarding chronic complications of diabetes mellitus**

A. Diabetic cardiomyopathy leads to diastolic dysfunction

B.   Diabetic nephropathy damage leads to acute renal failure.

C.   Diabetic neuropathy leads to diabetic foot.

D.   Diabetic retinopathy is a growth of friable and poor-quality new blood vessels in the retina as well as macular edema

E.   Macrovascular disease accelerates atherosclerosis

20.   Causes of obesity include:

A.   Genetic.

B.   Diet.

C.   Hypothyroidism.

D.   Hypothalamic surgery.

E.   Psychological.

9.1.b Questions with answers

1.   The following are statements regarding thyroid diseases:

T   A.   Thyroid carcinoma is more frequent in females than males.

F   B.   Lymphatic metastasis frequently occur in follicular thyroid carcinoma.

T   C.   Medullary thyroid carcinoma produces calcitonin.

T   D.   Atrial fiibrillation is a complication of thyrotoxicosis.

T   E.   Secondary hypercholesterolemia is a feature of hypothyroidism.

2.   The following are statements regarding thyroid diseases:

T   A.   Graves disease is more common in females.

F   B.   Hashimoto's thyroiditis is the most common cause of cretinism.

F   C.   In Graves disease, the thyroid gland is markedly enlarged and irregular.

T   D.   The most frequent cause of diffuse goitre is iodine deficiency.

T   E.   Compression on the trachea is a complication of multinodular goiter.

3.   The following are statements regarding Graves disease

F   A.   Blood levels of thyroid stimulating hormone (TSH) is elevated

T   B.   Heart failure is a complication

T   C.   Proptosis is one of its feature

T   D.   Basal metabolic rate is increased

F   E.   It frequently presents as a solitary thyroid nodule

4.   The following are statements regarding thyroid cancer

F   A.   It is rarely found in a euthyroid patient.

T   B.   Papillary thyroid cancer often found in young females

F   C.   Majority of cases are follicular thyroid cancer

F   D.   Anaplastic thyroid cancer is responsive well to treatment

T   E.   Fine needle aspiration is diagnostic

5.   The following are statements regarding papillary thyroid carcinoma

T   A.   It is the most common type of thyroid cancer

F   B.   it is more likely to invade blood vessels

T   C.   Orphan Annie eye nuclear inclusions are characteristic histological finding

F   D.   Chest x rays are commonly performed in diagnosis

T   E.   Thyroglobulin is used as a tumor marker for well-differentiated papillary thyroid cancer

6. **The following are statements regarding acromegaly**

F   A.   It is a syndrome that results when the anterior pituitary gland produces excess growth hormone before epiphyseal plate closure at puberty

F   B.   It is easy to diagnose in the early stages

T   C.   It is often associated with gigantism

T   D.   Hypertension is a complication

T   E.   Insulin-like growth factor 1 (IGF-1) provides the most sensitive lab test for the diagnosis of acromegaly

7. **Signs and symptoms of Cushing's syndrome include:**

F   A.   Weight loss

T   B.   irritability

T   C.   Muscle and bone weakness

T   D.   Diabetes mellitus

F   E.   Hypotension

8. **Causes of syndrome of inappropriate antidiuretic hormone secretion include:**

T   A.   Meningitis

T   B.   Subarachnoid hemorrhage

T   C.   Lung cancer

T D. Brain abscess

T E. Guillain-Barré syndrome

9. The following are statements regarding hypercalcaemia

T A. If caused by primary hyperparathyroidism, serum phosphate is low.

F B. Chronic renal failure is a common cause.

T C. There is polyuria.

T D. Renal stone formation is a complication.

F E. Medullary carcinoma of the thyroid is a cause.

10. The following are statements regarding adrenal diseases:

T A. Auto-immune disease is a cause of adrenal hypofunction.

T B. Hyperpigmentation occurs in primary adrenal failure.

T C. Adrenal insufficiency causes hyponatremia.

T D. Hypertension is a feature of Conn's syndrome.

F E. Pheochromocytoma causes hypotension.

11. The following are statements regarding pheochromocytoma

T A. It is a tumor of chromaffin cells that arises inside the adrenal glands

F B. Hypotention is a feature

F C. Men are likely to inherit the disease more than women

T D. This syndrome is mostly occur in between the ages of 30 to 60.

T E. Excess sweating is a presentation

12. The following are statements regarding hyperaldosteronism

F A. Most cases of primary hyperaldosteronism are caused by a cancerous tumor of the adrenal gland.

F B. The disease is common above age of 60

T C. Cirrhosis of the liver is a cause of secondary hyperaldosteronism

T D. Heart failure is a cause of secondary hyperaldosteronism

F E. High serum potassium is a symptom

13. Characteristic symptoms of Addison's crisis include:

T A. Sudden penetrating pain in the legs, lower back or abdomen

F B. Severe vomiting but without diarrhea

F C. Hyperglycemia

F D. Hypernatremia

F E. Hypocalcemia

14. Causes of Conn syndrome include:

T A. Adrenal carcinoma

F B. Adrenal hypoplasia

T C. Adrenal adenoma

T   D.   Dexamethasone-suppressible hyperaldosteronism

T   E.   Disorders of the renin-angiotensin system

15. Features of Cushing's syndrome include:

T   A.   Hypokalemia.

F   B.   Metabolic acidosis.

F   C.   Postural hypotension.

T   D.   Truncal obesity.

T   E.   Hirsutism.

16. The following are statements regarding diabetes mellitus (DM)

F   A.   Type 2 diabetes mellitus is characterized by loss of the insulin-producing beta cells of the islets of Langerhans in the pancreas

T   B.   Type 1 diabetes is of the immune-mediated nature

F   C.   Type 1 diabetes mellitus is characterized by insulin resistance

T   D.   Gestational diabetes mellitus resembles type 2 diabetes in several respects

T   E.   Prediabetes indicates a condition that occurs when a person's blood glucose levels are higher than normal but not high enough for a diagnosis of type 2 DM

17. The following are statements regarding diabetes mellitus:

F   A.   Type 2 diabetes is more common in children.

F   B.   Diagnosis is by measurement of HBA_{1c} level.

T   C.   Hyperthyroidism is a cause.

T   D.   Deposition of amyloid in the islet of Langerhans is seen in type 2 diabetes.

T   E.   Obesity is a predisposing factor for type 2 diabetes.

18. The following are statements regarding acute complications of diabetes mellitus

T   A.   Elevated levels of ketone bodies in the blood decrease the blood's pH leading to diabetic ketoacidosis

T   B.   Severe abdominal pain is common in diabetic ketoacidosis.

T   C.   Hyperosmolar nonketotic state is sharing many symptoms with diabetic ketoacidosis

T   D.   Electrolyte imbalances are common in hyperosmolar nonketotic

T   E.   The patient may become agitated, sweaty, weak in hypoglycemia

19. The following are statements regarding chronic complications of diabetes mellitus

T   A.   Diabetic cardiomyopathy leads to diastolic dysfunction

F   B.   Diabetic nephropathy damage leads to acute renal failure.

T   C.   Diabetic neuropathy leads to diabetic foot.

T   D.   Diabetic retinopathy is a growth of friable and poor-quality new blood vessels in the retina as well as macular edema

T   E.   Macrovascular disease accelerates atherosclerosis

20. Causes of obesity include:

T   A.   Genetic.

T   B.   Diet.

T   C.   Hypothyroidism.

T   D.   Hypothalamic surgery.

T   E.   Psychological.

9.2 Other Microbiology Related Topics

9.2.a Questions without answers

1. **The following are pairs regarding antibiotics and their main mechanisms of resistance:**

A.	Penicillin	:	Alteration of penicillin-binding proteins
B.	Aminoglycosides	:	Inactivating enzymes
C.	Tetracycline	:	Inactivating enzymes
D.	Chloramphenicol	:	Efflux pump
E.	Quinolones	:	Alteration in the DNA gyrase

2. **Methicillin-resistant *Staphylococcus aureus***

    A. has altered penicillin-binding proteins (PBPs).

    B. is resistant to oxacillin in the disc diffusion test.

    C. is catalase and coagulase negative.

    D. is commonly associated with nosocomial infections.

    E. is usually sensitive to cephalosporins.

3. **The following statements are regarding hospital infection and prevention:**

   A.   It does not include infection occurring 48 hours after discharge.

   B.   Antibiotic prophylaxis is indicated patients undergoing "clean surgery" to prevent post-operative wound sepsis.

   C.   Intravenous vancomycin should be given to nurses with methicillin-resistant *Staphylococcus aureus* (MRSA) nasal carriage.

   D.   ESBL-producing *Klebsiella* sp. is one of the important nosocomial pathogens.

   E.   Hospital staff with nasal carriage of MRSA is granted leave for a certain period.

4. **The following are the advantages and disadvantages of live and inactivated vaccines:**

	Live vaccines		**Inactivated vaccines**
A.	Antibody response consists of IgG and IgA.	:	Antibody response consists of IgG only.
B.	Cell-mediated immunity is poor.	:	Cell-mediated immunity is good.
C.	No reversion to virulence.	:	Reversion to virulence is common.
D.	Duration of immunity is short-term.	:	Duration of immunity is long-

term.

E.   Needs an adjuvant.   :   Do not need an
                                             adjuvant.

5.   Meningococcal vaccine

A.   induces a life-long immunity.

B.   does not contain capsular polysaccharide of *Neisseria meningitidis* serogroup B.

C.   is indicated in splenectomized individuals.

D.   is compulsory for Umrah and Hajj pilgrims to Mecca.

E.   is contraindicated in patients with terminal complement deficiencies.

6.   The following are statements regarding infections in febrile neutropenic patients:

A.   The risk of infection increases significantly if the neutrophil count falls below $0.5 \times 10^9/l$.

B.   The causative organisms are often derived from the patient's own flora.

C.   HEPA filters help to reduce the incidence of *Aspergillus* infection.

D.   Gut decontamination using non-absorbable antibiotics help in the prevention.

E.   If the patient remains febrile after an appropriate antibiotic therapy, amphotericin B should be added in the regimen.

7. **The following statements are regarding the role of normal flora in disease:**

    A. *Streptococcus mutans* is found in large numbers in dental plagues and dental caries.

    B. Pseudomembranous colitis is due to overgrowth of *Clostridium perfringens*.

    C. *Eikenella corrodens* causes soft tissue infections following human bites.

    D. Anaerobes in gingival crevices contribute to etiology of periodontal disease.

    E. Viridans streptococci causes infective endocarditis following dental extraction in patients with rheumatic heart disease.

8. **The following are statements regarding candidiasis:**

    A.
    It is almost always exogenous in origin.

    B.
    Candidal intertrigo, which presents with vesicles in the axillae, is commonly found in obese individuals.

    C. Chronic mucocutaneous candidiasis is often associated with B cell deficiency.

    D.
    Gram-stained smears of clinical specimens show presence of budding cells.

    E.
    Fluconazole can be used in the treatment.

9. **Kawasaki syndrome**

   A.   is an acute vasculitis primarily affecting the elderly.

   B.   is characterized by unresponsiveness to superantigen.

   C.   is associated with an increased risk of coronary artery disease.

   D.   presents with erythema and desquamation of palms and soles.

   E.   is treated with intravenous cloxacillin.

10. **The following are statements regarding dengue and other viral hemorrhagic fevers:**

   A.   Re-infection with a dengue virus of a different serotype after a primary attack may result in a milder disease.

   B.   Chikungunya hemorrhagic fever presents with sudden onset of biphasic fever and maculopapular rash.

   C.   Dengue and yellow fever viruses provide significant cross-immunity.

   D.   Dengue and Chikungunya hemorrhagic fever are both transmitted via bites of *Aedes aegypti*.

   E.   Korean hemorrhagic fever can be treated with ribavirin.

9.2.b Questions with answers

1. **The following are pairs regarding antibiotics and their main mechanisms of resistance:**

T A. Penicillin : Alteration of penicillin-binding proteins

T B. Aminoglycosides : Inactivating enzymes

F C. Tetracycline : Inactivating enzymes

F D. Chloramphenicol : Efflux pump

T E. Quinolones : Alteration in the DNA gyrase

2. **Methicillin-resistant *Staphylococcus aureus***

T A. has altered penicillin-binding proteins (PBPs).

T B. is resistant to oxacillin in the disc diffusion test.

F C. is catalase and coagulase negative.

T D. is commonly associated with nosocomial infections.

F E. is usually sensitive to cephalosporins.

3. **The following statements are regarding hospital infection and prevention:**

F   A.   It does not include infection occurring 48 hours after discharge.

F   B.   Antibiotic prophylaxis is indicated patients undergoing "clean surgery" to prevent post-operative wound sepsis.

F   C.   Intravenous vancomycin should be given to nurses with methicillin-resistant *Staphylococcus aureus* (MRSA) nasal carriage.

T   D.   ESBL-producing *Klebsiella* sp. is one of the important nosocomial pathogens.

T   E.   Hospital staff with nasal carriage of MRSA is granted leave for a certain period.

4.   **The following are the advantages and disadvantages of live and inactivated vaccines:**

		Live vaccines		**Inactivated vaccines**
T	A.	Antibody response consists of IgG and IgA.	:	Antibody response consists of IgG only.
F	B.	Cell-mediated immunity is poor.	:	Cell-mediated immunity is good.
F	C.	No reversion to virulence.	:	Reversion to virulence is common.
F	D.	Duration of immunity is short-term.	:	Duration of immunity is long-term.
F	E.	Needs an adjuvant.	:	Do not need an

adjuvant.

5.   Meningococcal vaccine

F   A.   induces a life-long immunity.

T   B.   does not contain capsular polysaccharide of *Neisseria meningitidis* serogroup B.

T   C.   is indicated in splenectomized individuals.

T   D.   is compulsory for Umrah and Hajj pilgrims to Mecca.

F   E.   is contraindicated in patients with terminal complement deficiencies.

6.   The following are statements regarding infections in febrile neutropenic patients:

T   A.   The risk of infection increases significantly if the neutrophil count falls below $0.5 \times 10^9/l$.

T   B.   The causative organisms are often derived from the patient's own flora.

T   C.   HEPA filters help to reduce the incidence of *Aspergillus* infection.

F   D.   Gut decontamination using non-absorbable antibiotics help in the prevention.

T   E.   If the patient remains febrile after an appropriate antibiotic therapy, amphotericin B should be added in the regimen.

7. **The following statements are regarding the role of normal flora in disease:**

T   A.   *Streptococcus mutans* is found in large numbers in dental plagues and dental caries.

F   B.   Pseudomembranous colitis is due to overgrowth of *Clostridium perfringens*.

T   C.   *Eikenella corrodens* causes soft tissue infections following human bites.

T   D.   Anaerobes in gingival crevices contribute to etiology of periodontal disease.

T   E.   Viridans streptococci causes infective endocarditis following dental extraction in patients with rheumatic heart disease.

8. **The following are statements regarding candidiasis:**

F   A.

It is almost always exogenous in origin.

T   B.

Candidal intertrigo, which presents with vesicles in the axillae, is commonly found in obese individuals.

F   C.   Chronic mucocutaneous candidiasis is often associated with B cell deficiency.

T   D.

Gram-stained smears of clinical specimens show presence of budding cells.

T   E.

Fluconazole can be used in the treatment.

9. **Kawasaki syndrome**

F   A.   is an acute vasculitis primarily affecting the elderly.

F   B.   is characterized by unresponsiveness to superantigen.

T   C.   is associated with an increased risk of coronary artery disease.

T   D.   presents with erythema and desquamation of palms and soles.

F   E.   is treated with intravenous cloxacillin.

10. The following are statements regarding dengue and other viral hemorrhagic fevers:

F   A.   Re-infection with a dengue virus of a different serotype after a primary attack may result in a milder disease.

T   B.   Chikungunya hemorrhagic fever presents with sudden onset of biphasic fever and maculopapular rash.

F   C.   Dengue and yellow fever viruses provide significant cross-immunity.

T   D.   Dengue and Chikungunya hemorrhagic fever are both transmitted via bites of *Aedes aegypti.*

T   E.   Korean hemorrhagic fever can be treated with ribavirin.

10 NERVOUS SYSTEM

10.1 Pathology of Nervous System

  10.1.a Questions without answers

1.   The following are statements regarding Parkinson's disease:

A.   It is characterized clinically by tremor

B.   The amyloid plaques are characteristic

C.   There are bradykinesia and rigidity

D.   Usually become manifest below the age of 45 years

E.   Lewy bodies are characteristic

2.   The following are statements regarding Parkinson's disease:

A.   Headache is the first presentation

B.   Lewy bodies are characteristic

C.   There is mask face presentation

D.   It is rarely caused dementia.

E.   Occurrence of infections at the late stage of disease.

3.   **The characteristic histological changes in Alzheimer's disease include:**

A.   Amyloid plaques

B.   Neurofibrillary tangles

C.   Neuronal loss

D.   Granulomatous inflammation

E.   Perivascular amyloid

4.   **The following are statements regarding demyelinating disorders**

A.   Affect myelin and interrupt nerve transmission

B.   Symptoms reflect deficits in any part of the nervous system.

C.   Multiple sclerosis is inherited disorder.

D.   Leukodystrophies mean primary demyelination

E.   In acquired type, the normally formed myelin is injured.

5.   **The following are statements regarding multiple sclerosis (MS)**

A.   It is the most common demyelinating disease that affects brain and spinal cord.

B.   It affects men more than women.

C. It is characterized by the presence of multiple areas of demyelination, termed plaques.

D. Magnetic Resonance Imaging (MRI scan) is not a diagnostic tool .

E. The external appearance of the brain and spinal cord is usually normal.

6. **The following are statements regarding subacute combined degeneration (SCD)**

A. It is a progressive disorder that is due to vitamin B6 deficiency.

B. In this disorder, the columns of sensory nerve fibers in the spinal cord degenerate.

C. In this disorder, rarely, dementia develops.

D. The disorder begins with a general feeling of weakness.

E. The diagnosis is made based on histopathology specimen.

7. **The following are statements regarding Wernicke-Korsakoff Syndrome:**

A. The cause of the disease is malnutrition, especially lack of vitamin B12.

B. It is characterized by fairly rapid onset of confusion, paralysia of exterocular muscles and ataxia.

C. Korsakoff psychosis , is a permanent memory deficit occur if the wernicke-korsakoff syndrom is not treated well.

D. Wernicke's encephalopathy involves damage to multiple nerves in the brain, spinal cord and the peripheral nervous system.

E. Clinically there are vision changes

8. **Characteristic features of glioblastoma multiforme include:**

A. Evidence of astrocytic differentiation

B. Perivascular pseudorosette formation

C. Cellular pleomorphism

D. Mitotic activity

E. Microvascular proliferation

9. **The characteristic histologic features of pilocytic astrocytoma include:**

A. Hair-like cell processes

B. Rosenthal fibers

C. Homer Wright rosettes

D. Ependymal rosettes

E. Hyaline granular bodies

10. **The following are statements regarding medullosblastoma**

A. It is derived from neuronal cells.

B. It occurs predominantly in children.

C. It is located mostly in the cerebral cortex.

D. It spreads via the lymphatic pathway.

E.   It is a slow malignant tumor.

11.   Complications of cerebral abscesses include:

A.   Meningitis

B.   Intracranial herniation

C.   Focal neurological deficit

D.   Tumor

E.   Epilepsy

12.   Cerebrospinal fluid findings in bacterial meningitis include:

A.   Increased lymphocytes

B.   Low glucose

C.   Low protein

D.   Decrease pressure

E.   Increase turbidity

13.   Effects of rapidly progressing hydrocephalus include:

A.   Tachycardia

B.   Papilloedema

C.   Decrease consciousness

D.   Increase in head size in adults

E.   Headache

14. **The following are statements regarding communicating hydrocephalus**

    A. It is due to degeneration of brain substance

    B. Dandy walker syndrome is one of the cause

    C. Hydrocephalus ex-vacuo is an example

    D. Tonsillar herniation in one of the complications

    E. Papilloedema is present in chronic cases

15. **Causes of subarachnoid hemorrhage include:**

    A. Bleeding in a ventricle

    B. Rupture of bridging veins

    C. Vascular malformation

    D. Rupture of berry aneurysm

    E. Rupture of middle meningeal artery

16. **The following are statements regarding intracranial haemorrhage**

    A. Lead to increase intracranial pressure

    B. Bleeding from the artery is self limited

    C. Ruptured aneurysm is the main cause of subdural hematoma

    D. Arterial injury seen in Shaken baby syndrome

    E. Patient on anticoagulant has high risk

17. **Causes of increased intracranial pressure include:**

   A.   Acute liver failure

   B.   Hypertension

   C.   Heart failure

   D.   Urinary stone

   E.   Coughing

18. **Intracranial pressure is increased due to**

   A.   decreased production of CSF

   B.   cerebral tumors

   C.   subarachnoid hemorrhage

   D.   spinal cord infarction

   E.   epidural hematoma.

19. **Complications of increased intracranial pressure include:**

   A.   Papilloedema

   B.   Hydrocephalus

   C.   Constricted pupils

   D.   Fracture of skull bone

   E.   Damage to intracranial nerves

20. **The following are statements regarding Huntington's disease**

A. It affects muscle coordination and leads to cognitive decline and psychiatric problems

B. It typically becomes noticeable in mid-adult life

C. It is the rare common genetic cause of abnormal involuntary writhing movements called chorea

D. It is much more common in people of Asia or Africa than in those of Western European descent

E. The disease is caused by an autosomal dominant mutation.

10.1.b Questions with answers

1.   The following are statements regarding Parkinson's disease:

T   A.   It is characterized clinically by tremor

F   B.   The amyloid plaques are characteristic

T   C.   There are bradykinesia and rigidity

F   D.   Usually become manifest below the age of 45 years

T   E.   Lewy bodies are characteristic

2.   The following are statements regarding Parkinson's disease:

F   A.   Headache is the first presentation

T   B.   Lewy bodies are characteristic

T   C.   There is mask face presentation

F   D.   It is rarely caused dementia.

T   E.   Occurrence of infections at the late stage of disease.

3.   The characteristic histological changes in Alzheimer's disease include:

T   A.   Amyloid plaques

T   B.   Neurofibrillary tangles

T   C.   Neuronal loss

F   D.   Granulomatous inflammation

T   E.   Perivascular amyloid

4.   **The following are statements regarding demyelinating disorders**

T   A.   Affect myelin and interrupt nerve transmission

T   B.   Symptoms reflect deficits in any part of the nervous system.

F   C.   Multiple sclerosis is inherited disorder.

T   D.   Leukodystrophies mean primary demyelination

T   E.   In acquired type, the normally formed myelin is injured.

5.   **The following are statements regarding multiple sclerosis (MS)**

T   A.   It is the most common demyelinating disease that affects brain and spinal cord.

F   B.   It affects men more than women.

T   C.   It is characterized by the presence of multiple areas of demyelination, termed plaques.

F   D.   Magnetic Resonance Imaging (MRI scan) is not a diagnostic tool .

T   E.   The external appearance of the brain and spinal cord is usually normal.

6.   **The following are statements regarding subacute combined degeneration (SCD)**

F   A.   It is a progressive disorder that is due to vitamin B6 deficiency.

T   B.   In this disorder, the columns of sensory nerve fibers in the spinal cord degenerate.

T   C.   In this disorder, rarely, dementia develops.

T   D.   The disorder begins with a general feeling of weakness.

F   E.   The diagnosis is made based on histopathology specimen.

7. The following are statements regarding Wernicke-Korsakoff Syndrome:

F   A.   The cause of the disease is malnutrition, especially lack of vitamin B12.

T   B.   It is characterized by fairly rapid onset of confusion, paralysia of exterocular muscles and ataxia.

T   C.   Korsakoff psychosis , is a permanent memory deficit occur if the wernicke-korsakoff syndrom is not treated well.

T   D.   Wernicke's encephalopathy involves damage to multiple nerves in the brain, spinal cord and the peripheral nervous system.

T   E.   Clinically there are vision changes

8. Characteristic features of glioblastoma multiforme include:

T   A.   Evidence of astrocytic differentiation

F   B.   Perivascular pseudorosette formation

T   C.   Cellular pleomorphism

T   D.   Mitotic activity

T   E.   Microvascular proliferation

9.   The characteristic histologic features of pilocytic astrocytoma include:

T   A.   Hair-like cell processes

T   B.   Rosenthal fibers

F   C.   Homer Wright rosettes

F   D.   Ependymal rosettes

T   E.   Hyaline granular bodies

10.   The following are statements regarding medullosblastoma

F   A.   It is derived from neuronal cells.

T   B.   It occurs predominantly in children.

F   C.   It is located mostly in the cerebral cortex.

F   D.   It spreads via the lymphatic pathway.

F   E.   It is a slow malignant tumor.

11.   Complications of cerebral abscesses include:

T   A.   Meningitis

T   B.   Intracranial herniation

T   C.   Focal neurological deficit

F   D.   Tumor

T   E.   Epilepsy

12.   **Cerebrospinal fluid findings in bacterial meningitis include:**

F   A.   Increased lymphocytes

T   B.   Low glucose

F   C.   Low protein

F   D.   Decrease pressure

T   E.   Increase turbidity

13.   **Effects of rapidly progressing hydrocephalus include:**

F   A.   Tachycardia

T   B.   Papilloedema

T   C.   Decrease consciousness

F   D.   Increase in head size in adults

T   E.   Headache

14.   **The following are statements regarding communicating hydrocephalus**

F   A.   It is due to degeneration of brain substance

F   B.   Dandy walker syndrome is one of the cause

F   C.   Hydrocephalus ex-vacuo is an example

T   D.   Tonsillar herniation in one of the complications

F   E.   Papilloedema is present in chronic cases

15.   Causes of subarachnoid hemorrhage include:

T   A.   Bleeding in a ventricle

F   B.   Rupture of bridging veins

T   C.   Vascular malformation

T   D.   Rupture of berry aneurysm

F   E.   Rupture of middle meningeal artery

16.   The following are statements regarding intracranial haemorrhage

T   A.   Lead to increase intracranial pressure

F   B.   Bleeding from the artery is self limited

F   C.   Ruptured aneurysm is the main cause of subdural hematoma

F   D.   Arterial injury seen in Shaken baby syndrome

T   E.   Patient on anticoagulant has high risk

17.   Causes of increased intracranial pressure include:

T   A.   Acute liver failure

T   B.   Hypertension

F   C.   Heart failure

F   D.   Urinary stone

T   E.   Coughing

18.   Intracranial pressure is increased due to

F   A.   decreased production of CSF

T   B.   cerebral tumors

T   C.   subarachnoid hemorrhage

F   D.   spinal cord infarction

T   E.   epidural hematoma.

19.   Complications of increased intracranial pressure include:

T   A.   Papilloedema

T   B.   Hydrocephalus

F   C.   Constricted pupils

F   D.   Fracture of skull bone

T   E.   Damage to intracranial nerves

20.   The following are statements regarding Huntington's disease

T   A.   It affects muscle coordination and leads to cognitive decline and psychiatric problems

T   B.   It typically becomes noticeable in mid-adult life

F   C.   It is the rare common genetic cause of abnormal involuntary writhing movements called chorea

F   D.   It is much more common in people of Asia or Africa than in those of Western European descent

T   E.   The disease is caused by an autosomal dominant mutation.

10.2 Microbiology of Nervous System

10.2.a Questions without answers

1.   A 45-year-old man, an intravenous drug user, presented with low grade fever and mild headache for one week. Physical examination revealed neck rigidity. India ink preparation of CSF showed encapsulated yeasts. The following are statements regarding the case:

    A.   The likely causative organism is *Candida albicans*.

    B.   AIDS may be considered as one of the underlying conditions.

    C.   Hematogenous spread of the causative organism from the lungs is likely.

    D.   The causative organism does not grow on artificial media.

    E.   He should be treated with amphotericin B and 5-flucytosine.

2.   The following are statements regarding bacterial meningitis:

A. Neonatal meningitis is commonly caused by *Streptococcus pneumoniae*.

B. Latex agglutination test helps in diagnosis of partially-treated meningitis.

C. Ciprofloxacin is given to household contacts of an index case of meningococcal meningitis.

D. Reduced protein but raised glucose levels are detected in cerebrospinal fluid.

E. *Haemophilus influenzae* meningitis can be prevented by a polysaccharide vaccine.

3. **The following are statements regarding laboratory diagnosis of meningitis:**

A. Blood culture is one of the important specimens to be taken.

B. In bacterial meningitis, glucose level in cerebrospinal fluid (CSF) is higher than that in plasma.

C. In viral meningitis, CSF protein is raised but glucose is within normal limits.

D. CSF cytology shows predominance of polymorphs in tuberculous meningitis.

E. Latex agglutination test detects *Haemophilus influenzae* antigen in CSF.

4. **A 45-year-old lady presented with high grade fever, severe headache and cough productive of purulent sputum. There was neck rigidity. Gram-stained smear of her cerebrospinal fluid revealed numerous polymorphs and**

Gram-positive diplococci. The following are statements regarding the case:

A.   The causative organism is likely to be resistant to optochin.

B.   *Streptococcus penumoniae* should be considered as one of the causative organisms.

C.   Cerebrospinal fluid biochemistry shows low glucose and high protein levels.

D.   Aminoglycoside is the antibiotic of choice in the treatment.

E.   Polysaccharide vaccine is available for its prevention.

5.   Poliomyelitis

A.   is an enteroviral infection.

B.   has an extremely long incubation period.

C.   is characterized by damage and death of the anterior horn cells.

D.   almost always presents with paralysis.

E.   can be prevented by an oral vaccine.

10.2.b Questions with answers

1. **A 45-year-old man, an intravenous drug user, presented with low grade fever and mild headache for one week. Physical examination revealed neck rigidity. India ink preparation of CSF showed encapsulated yeasts. The following are statements regarding the case:**

F   A.   The likely causative organism is *Candida albicans*.

T   B.   AIDS may be considered as one of the underlying conditions.

T   C.   Hematogenous spread of the causative organism from the lungs is likely.

F   D.   The causative organism does not grow on artificial media.

T   E.   He should be treated with amphotericin B and 5-flucytosine.

2. **The following are statements regarding bacterial meningitis:**

F   A.   Neonatal meningitis is commonly caused by *Streptococcus pneumoniae*.

T   B.   Latex agglutination test helps in diagnosis of partially-treated meningitis.

T   C.   Ciprofloxacin is given to household contacts of an index case of meningococcal meningitis.

F   D.   Reduced protein but raised glucose levels are detected in cerebrospinal fluid.

T   E.   *Haemophilus influenzae* meningitis can be prevented by a polysaccharide vaccine.

3. The following are statements regarding laboratory diagnosis of meningitis:

T   A.   Blood culture is one of the important specimens to be taken.

F   B.   In bacterial meningitis, glucose level in cerebrospinal fluid (CSF) is higher than that in plasma.

T   C.   In viral meningitis, CSF protein is raised but glucose is within normal limits.

F   D.   CSF cytology shows predominance of polymorphs in tuberculous meningitis.

T   E.   Latex agglutination test detects *Haemophilus influenzae* antigen in CSF.

4. A 45-year-old lady presented with high grade fever, severe headache and cough productive of purulent sputum. There was neck rigidity. Gram-stained smear of her cerebrospinal fluid revealed numerous polymorphs and Gram-positive diplococci. The following are statements regarding the case:

F   A.   The causative organism is likely to be resistant to optochin.

T   B.   *Streptococcus penumoniae* should be considered as one of the causative organisms.

T   C.   Cerebrospinal fluid biochemistry shows low glucose and high protein levels.

F   D.   Aminoglycoside is the antibiotic of choice in the treatment.

T   E.   Polysaccharide vaccine is available for its prevention.

5.   Poliomyelitis

T   A.   is an enteroviral infection.

F   B.   has an extremely long incubation period.

T   C.   is characterized by damage and death of the anterior horn cells.

F   D.   almost always presents with paralysis.

T   E.   can be prevented by an oral vaccine.

ABOUT THE AUTHORS

Dr. Muhamed T. Osman; PhD, presently, is Associate Professor of Pathology in Faculty of Medicine and Defence Health, National Defence University of Malaysia. He was Consultant Pathologist and Clinical Lecturer at Teaching Laboratories of Medical City in Baghdad, Iraq and Senior Lecturer of Pathology at UiTM Malaysia. He is the author of six books and has published more than 60 papers in peer reviewed journals.

Dr. Sabiha Pit; FRCPath, presently is Professor of Medical Microbiology in Faculty of Medicine and Defence Health, National Defence University of Malaysia. She has held the post of Professor of Medical Microbiology in Universiti Teknologi MARA (UiTM) and MAHSA University, Malaysia. She is the author of three books and has published more than 60 papers in peer reviewed journals.

www.ingramcontent.com/pod-product-compliance
Lightning Source LLC
Chambersburg PA
CBHW051441170526
45166CB00001B/68